WILLIAMS-SONOMA
COLLECTION

HEALTHY
SIDE
DISHES

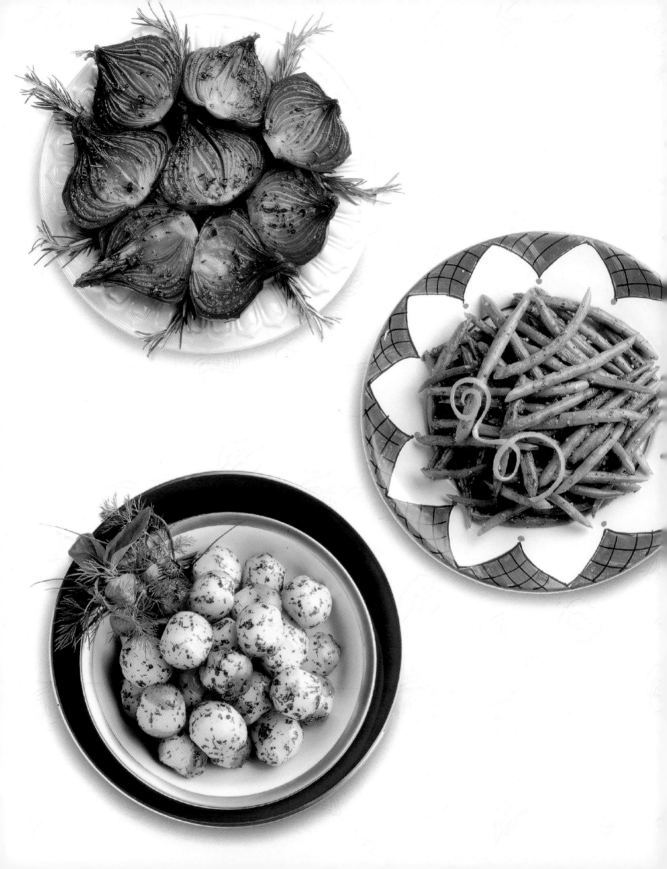

WILLIAMS-SONOMA
COLLECTION

HEALTHY SIDE DISHES

GENERAL EDITOR

CHUCK WILLIAMS

RECIPES BY

DIANE ROSSEN WORTHINGTON

PHOTOGRAPHY BY

ALLAN ROSENBERG & ALLEN V. LOTT

TIME
LIFE
BOOKS

**Time-Life Books is a division of
Time-Life Incorporated**

President & CEO: John Fahey, Jr.

TIME-LIFE BOOKS

President, Time-Life Books: John D. Hall
Vice President & Publisher: Terry Newell
Director of New Product Development: Regina Hall
Director of Financial Operations: J. Brian Birky
Editorial Director: Donia Ann Steele

WILLIAMS-SONOMA
Founder: Chuck Williams

WELDON OWEN INC.
President: John Owen
Publisher/Vice President: Wendely Harvey
Associate Publisher: Tori Ritchie
Project Coordinator: Jill Fox
Consulting Editor: Norman Kolpas
Recipe Analysis & Nutritional Consultation:
    Hill Nutrition Associates Inc.
    Lynne S. Hill, MS, RD; William A. Hill, MS, RD
Copy Editor: Sharon Silva
Art Director: John Bull
Designer: Patty Hill
Production Director: Stephanie Sherman
Production Editor: Janique Gascoigne
Co-Editions Director: Derek Barton
Co-Editions Production Manager: Tarji Mickelson
Food & Prop Stylist: Heidi Gintner
Associate Food & Prop Stylist: Danielle Di Salvo
Assistant Food Stylist: Nette Scott
Props Courtesy: Sandra Griswold
Indexer: ALTA Indexing Service
Proofreaders: Ken DellaPenta, Desne Border
Illustrator: Diana Reiss-Koncar
Special Thanks: Claire Sanchez, Marguerite Ozburn,
    Jennifer Mullins, Mick Bagnato

The Williams-Sonoma Healthy Collection
conceived & produced by Weldon Owen Inc.
814 Montgomery Street, San Francisco, CA 94133

In collaboration with Williams-Sonoma
100 North Point, San Francisco, CA 94133

Production by Mandarin Offset, Hong Kong
Printed in China

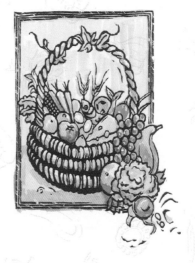

A Weldon Owen Production

Copyright © 1995 Weldon Owen Inc.

Library of Congress
Cataloging-in-Publication Data:

Worthington, Diane Rossen.
    Healthy side dishes / general editor, Chuck Williams ;
recipes by Diane Rossen Worthington ; photography by
Allan Rosenberg & Allen V. Lott.
        p.   cm. — (Williams-Sonoma collection)
    "A Weldon Owen production"—T.p. verso.
    Includes index.
    ISBN 0-7835-4601-7
    1. Side dishes (Cookery)   2. Cookery (Vegetables)
3. Cookery (Rice)   4. Nutrition   5. Salt-free diet—Recipes.
I. Williams, Chuck.   II. Title.   III. Series.
TX801.W668 1995
641.8'1—dc20   95-10209
                                    CIP

*Cover: Side dishes offer an opportunity to serve unusual
ingredients in creative ways, such as colorful Tricolored Pepper
Sauté (recipe on page 16). Back Cover: Orange-Glazed Sweet
Potatoes (recipe on page 85) are a vitamin-packed, sweet treat.*

HEALTHY
SIDE
DISHES

CONTENTS

THE BASICS 6

VEGETABLES 14

POTATOES 76

RICE, BEANS & GRAINS 98

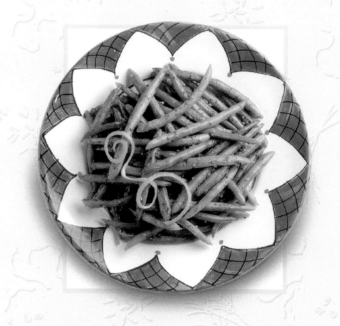

THE BASICS

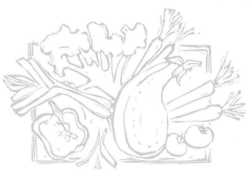

The point of the side dish recipes and health information in this book is to provide balanced meals without giving up any of the pleasures of eating. While not intended as a weight-loss guide, this book offers abundant inspiration, recipes and nutritional analysis tailored to designing a healthy eating style. A consensus of experts agree that a good diet is one in which 30 percent or fewer calories come from fat, about 15 percent from protein and about 55 percent from complex carbohydrates and one that is high in fiber and low in cholesterol and added salt. More than that, the ideal diet utilizes a variety of ingredients cooked in creative ways. The side dish recipes in this book feature seasonal vegetables, potatoes, rice, beans and grains in tempting combinations and use simple cooking techniques that bring out the food's flavor without adding fat and calories. This chapter begins where a good diet should begin, with a guide to properly selecting and storing the wonderful ingredients used in the recipes that make up *Healthy Side Dishes.*

COOKING HEALTHY SIDE DISHES

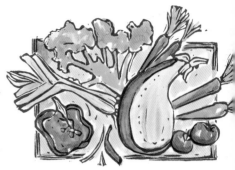

Establishing and maintaining a healthy diet doesn't usually take a revolutionary lifestyle change. Common sense can be your guide. Along with moderating sugar and alcohol intake, the key is to cook, serve and eat balanced meals. While in the past this balance was heavily weighted to main dish animal protein, today's guidelines suggest that dishes featuring vegetables and starches occupy a proportionately larger portion of the meal. The next step is to choose healthy recipes that utilize seasonal ingredients, are cooked using simple techniques that do not add fat (see below), are flavored without unnecessary sodium and are garnished for plenty of plate appeal.

Side dish hardly does justice to the role this part of the menu can play in eating well. Vegetables of every color, shape, texture and flavor, along with potato, rice, bean and grain dishes, offer a bountiful harvest of vitamins, minerals, complex carbohydrates and dietary fiber. Current medical research indicates some vegetables contain compounds thought to reduce the susceptibility to cancer while others possess elements that aid in lowering blood-cholesterol levels. Most importantly, side dishes provide the delightful variety necessary for well-rounded nutrition and satisfied appetites.

COOKING IT SIMPLY

Quick, simple cooking highlights the fresh tastes and textures of seasonal vegetables while helping to preserve their nutrients. To achieve the best results, follow these simple guidelines for the most common cooking methods. In any case, pay careful attention to the cooking time given in any particular recipe to achieve the desired results—whether crisp to the bite or soft enough to purée. To test any vegetable for doneness, insert a sharp knife tip or fork into the vegetable or remove a sample from the cooking vessel, blow on it to cool it and take a bite.

BOILING

Take care to select a pan large enough to hold the vegetables comfortably and allow for plenty of boiling water to circulate around them. Fill the pan with water and bring to a boil, add the vegetables and continue boiling until tender-crisp if they will be served in pieces or softer if they are to be puréed.

GRILLING OR BROILING

Prepare a fire in a charcoal grill or a gas barbecue or preheat an indoor broiler (griller). Away from the fire, coat the grill rack with nonstick cooking spray. When the coals or broiler are hot, arrange the vegetables on the grill rack or broiler (griller) pan and cook 3–4 inches (7.5–10 cm) away from the heat until tender and nicely browned, 3–6 minutes per side depending on the vegetable.

MICROWAVING

As an alternative to boiling or steaming vegetables, some cooks prefer to cook them in the microwave—although, because the vegetables tend to cook quickly, the timing can be harder to judge properly. Put the vegetables in a microwave-safe container, add about 2 tablespoons water, cover the container with its lid or microwave-proof plastic wrap and cook on the "high" setting until done, following manufacturer's instructions (times will vary with the power of the oven). Remove the lid or plastic wrap *very carefully* from the far side of the container, letting the steam escape away from you to avoid any burns.

Making healthy choices

Use side dishes to try unusual ingredients and to experiment with new ways of cooking. The first step in cooking healthy side dishes is to learn to choose, store and use the best ingredients possible.

Choosing Vegetables

The benefits of eating vegetables are as great as the choices available. Let variety be the byword of incorporating vegetables into a healthy diet, utilizing different vegetables daily. In general, for a well-balanced diet provide three to five 1-cup (8-oz/250-g) raw, leafy vegetable or fruit servings or ½-cup (4-oz/125-g) other vegetable servings per person, per day.

Growing interest in the health benefits and culinary pleasures of vegetables have been recognized by businesses. Large food stores have increased the dimensions of produce sections and old-fashioned farmer's markets are popular weekend haunts in big cities and small towns. Although it is tempting to purchase large quantities when faced with such abundance, most vegetables retain their vitamin and mineral content only a few days after harvest. Allowing for distribution time, purchase only about 3 days worth of vegetables at any time.

While modern shipping methods make it possible to find produce varieties all year round, the best nutrition and price is found in seasonal produce (see page 10). Use fresh items whenever possible, substituting frozen versions only when necessary.

Once purchased, fresh, seasonal produce must be properly stored for maximum nutrition and minimal waste. Moisture is the enemy of vegetable storage. For leafy vegetables, wash and completely dry all items as soon as possible after purchase. Even vegetables that will be peeled should be washed to prevent the transfer of harmful residue to the edible portion during preparation. In most cases, enclose dried vegetables in plastic containers designed for storage or in plastic bags. However, do not seal the plastic bags, so that air can circulate. To absorb any excess moisture, put a paper towel in the bottom of the container. Place the vegetables in the coldest part of the refrigerator until needed. Check vegetables daily and remove and discard moldy items.

SAUTÉING

For quick cooking on top of the stove, select a sauté pan or a wide frying pan with sloping sides that allow moisture to escape. Heat a thin film of oil in the pan over medium heat or heat the pan and, away from the fire, coat with nonstick cooking spray. Add the vegetables and stir frequently until done.

STEAMING

To assemble a steamer, place a steaming rack inside a saucepan so that it fits snugly. Add water to just below the bottom of the rack, then lay the vegetables on the rack. Cover and bring to a boil, steaming the vegetables to the desired degree of doneness. Or use a 2-piece steaming pot made for this purpose.

STIR-FRYING

To stir-fry Chinese-style in a wok or deep frying pan, heat a thin film of oil over medium-high heat or heat the pan first and, away from the fire, coat with nonstick cooking spray. Add the vegetables and, using a large spatula or spoon, stir constantly until done.

Use this guide to choose and store the most common produce. Basic preparation methods for these and other ingredients featured in the recipes in this book begin on page 120.

BEETS
Available from early spring to mid-summer, beets (beetroots) should be firm, smooth and dark red in color. Purchase with their greens attached, which is a sign of freshness. Store in the refrigerator. Raw beets yield about 55 calories per cup (5 oz/155 g) and are good sources of folate, magnesium, potassium and other minerals.

BELL PEPPERS
Whether red, yellow, green, orange or purple, bell peppers (capsicums) should have bright, deep color; firm, smooth, shiny surfaces and firm stems. Green ones are available year-round; others are seasonal. Store in plastic in the refrigerator. Rich in vitamin C and fiber—as well as vitamin A in red and yellow varieties—one medium pepper yields less than 20 calories.

BROCCOLI
Available year-round. Select broccoli that appears firm and bright green with compact, dark-green florets. Store in the refrigerator. There are about 45 calories in 1 cup (4 oz/125 g) of cooked broccoli, with lots of vitamin C and ample vitamin A, as well as iron, potassium and other minerals.

CARROTS
Available year-round. Carrots are best when firm, smooth and bright orange with attached greens. Store in the refrigerator. There are less than 70 calories in 1 cup (5 oz/155 g) of cooked carrots and they are an outstanding source of vitamin A, along with some vitamin C and various minerals.

EGGPLANTS
Available year-round. Eggplants (aubergines) should have glossy purple-black skins and bright green caps and feel heavy for their size. Raw eggplants yield about 30 calories per cup (5 oz/155 g) and provide some folate and potassium.

LEEKS
Available year-round. These members of the onion family should have firm white bulb ends and flexible, fresh-looking green stalks. Store in plastic in the refrigerator. A source of calcium, other minerals and vitamin C, raw leeks provide about 32 calories per cup (4 oz/125 g).

SPINACH
Available year-round. Select spinach with crisp, dark-green leaves, free of any soft spots or moisture. Store in plastic in the refrigerator. A source of vitamin A and minerals, 1 cup (7 oz/220 g) of cooked spinach yields about 40 calories.

SQUASHES
Available during the warm months of mid-spring to early autumn, summer squashes—most notably zucchini (courgette) and yellow summer squash—should feel firm and have blemish-free, brightly colored skins. Store in the refrigerator. A good source of vitamin A and minerals, cooked summer squashes yield about 36 calories per cup (5 oz/155 g).

Hard-shelled winter squashes, such as acorn, butternut and spaghetti squash, are available from early autumn to early winter. Choose those that feel heavy for their size, have good color, are firm and blemish-free. Store in a cool, dry place. Winter squashes are excellent sources of vitamin A, and, when cooked, average about 80 calories per cup (5 oz/155 g).

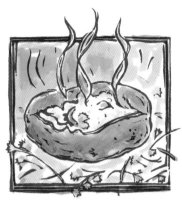

CHOOSING POTATOES

Although part of the vegetable world, potatoes stand in a class by themselves. The favored culinary staple of many meals, they put on the plate ample amounts of vitamin C, vitamin B6, iron, potassium and other minerals, all wrapped in a virtually fat-free package rich in complex carbohydrates and dietary fiber.

When selecting any kind of potato, choose those that are well-shaped, firm and free of blemishes, bruises and discolorations. Beware of those with green spots, indicating the presence of a toxic alkaloid called solanine that results from exposure to light. Potato sprouts or eyes are not harmful, although they increase peeling time and waste. Eyes may also indicate age. The older a potato, the higher the starch content. High-starch potatoes have less moisture and absorb other flavors well. Low-starch potatoes are more moist and hold their shape better after cooking. Make sure that small raw potatoes are truly "new" potatoes by gently rubbing their skins, which, being immature, should come off easily.

Do not wash potatoes before storing. Place most varieties in a vegetable bin or wrap them loosely in brown paper and store in a cool, dark place. Avoid plastic bags, which will trap moisture. New and waxy potatoes should be refrigerated. Cook most potatoes within 10 days of purchase, but new potatoes within 2–3 days.

Dozens of potato varieties exist but most can be classified under the following basic categories:

BAKING POTATOES

Also known as russet or Idaho potatoes, these large potatoes have thick brown skins. Their dry, mealy texture when cooked make them ideal for baking or mashing.

NEW POTATOES

Any kind of potato harvested in early summer, when small and immature is "new." The more tender, sweeter flesh is best enjoyed when steamed, boiled or roasted. Store in the refrigerator.

RED POTATOES

Red skinned potatoes with crisp, waxy, white flesh are best suited to steaming, boiling or roasting. Store in the refrigerator.

SWEET POTATOES & YAMS

A tuberous root vegetable unrelated to the potato, sweet potatoes have light to deep-red skin and sweet yellow flesh. They are an exceptionally good source of vitamins A, B and C.

Yams are tuberous root vegetables native to Africa with orange flesh. Although the taste and texture of sweet potatoes and yams are different, they can be used interchangeably in recipes.

WHITE POTATOES

These medium-sized potatoes have thin tan skins. When cooked, their textures are finer than baking varieties but coarser than waxy yellow potatoes, making them a good all-purpose choice.

YELLOW POTATOES

Varieties with thin skins and yellowish, waxy flesh are best used for steaming, boiling, roasting or sautéing. Store in the refrigerator.

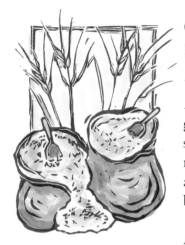

CHOOSING RICE, BEANS & GRAINS

High in dietary fiber, low in fat and free of cholesterol, grains and beans make exceptionally good side dish choices. They also offer generous amounts of protein, but, unlike animal proteins, no single plant source contains all nine of the essential amino acids needed for good nutrition. While this is not an important consideration where side dishes are concerned, when served as a main dish, they must be eaten in combinations (such as rice and beans together) to form complete proteins.

Rice provides basic sustenance for half the world's population. Among the many varieties of rice, the most popular are long-grain white rices. Some of the most flavorful varieties of white rice are basmati and jasmine. Brown rice is less processed than white rice. Because the bran is retained, brown rice is more nutritious than white rice but takes longer to cook. Wild rice is not a rice at all, but an aquatic grass that looks and cooks much like real rice. It has a nutty flavor that most people prefer mixed with white or brown rice into pilaf side dishes. Most types of rice are available in packages or bulk. Store all types of rice in tightly covered containers in a cool, dark place indefinitely.

Store other whole grains in tightly covered containers in the refrigerator for up to 5 months or at room temperature for up to 1 month. To protect grains from insects, add a few bay leaves to the container.

When purchasing beans, look for bright colors and uniform size; different sizes require different cooking times. Store beans in tightly covered glass containers in a cool, dark place and use within a year. The longer a bean has been stored, the longer it will take to cook.

TYPE OF RICE, BEAN OR GRAIN

1 Cup Cooked	Calories	Protein (g)	Fat (g)	Carbohydrate (g)
Rice 1 Cup (7 oz/220 g)				
Brown	220	4.6	1.6	46.0
Long-Grain White	264	5.5	0.6	57.0
Wild	166	6.5	0.6	35.0
Beans 1 Cup (7 oz/220 g)				
Beans, Black	227	15.2	0.9	40.7
Beans, White	249	17.4	0.6	44.9
Lentils	231	17.9	0.7	39.8
Pasta 1 Cup (3½ oz/105 g)	197	6.7	0.9	40.0
Polenta 1 Cup (6 oz/185 g)	146	3.4	0.4	31.4

READING A NUTRITIONAL CHART

Each recipe in this book has been evaluated by a registered dietitian. Beside each recipe, a chart similar to the one below lists the nutrient breakdown per serving. Use these numbers as a tool when putting together meals—and weeks and months of meals—designed for healthy eating.

All ingredients listed within each recipe have been included in the nutritional analysis. Exceptions are any items listed as "optional" and those added "to taste." When seasoning with salt, bear in mind that you are adding 2,200 mg of sodium for each teaspoon of regular salt and 1,800 mg per teaspoon of coarse kosher or sea salt. The addition of black or white pepper does not alter nutrient values. Substituted ingredients and accompaniments suggested in recipe introductions or shown in photographs have not been included in the analyses.

Quantities are based on a single serving of each recipe.

Protein, one of the basic life-giving nutrients, helps build and repair body tissues and performs other essential functions. One gram of protein contains 4 calories. A healthy diet derives about 15% of daily calories from protein.

Total fat is a measure of the grams of fat present in a serving, with 1 gram of fat equivalent to 9 calories (more than twice the calories in a gram of protein or carbohydrate). Experts recommend that fat intake be limited to a maximum 30% of total calories.

Cholesterol is present in foods of animal origin. Experts suggest a daily intake of no more than 300 mg. Plant foods contain no cholesterol.

Sodium, derived from salt and naturally present in many foods, helps maintain a proper balance of body fluids. Excess intake can lead to high blood pressure or hypertension in sodium-sensitive people. Those not sensitive should limit intake to about 2,400 mg daily.

Nutritional Analysis Per Serving:

CALORIES 34
(KILOJOULES 144)
PROTEIN 0 G
CARBOHYDRATES 3 G
TOTAL FAT 2 G
SATURATED FAT 0 G
CHOLESTEROL 0 MG
SODIUM 91 MG
DIETARY FIBER 1 G

Calories (kilojoules) provide a measure of the energy provided by any given food. A calorie equals the heat energy necessary to raise the temperature of 1 kg of water by 1° Celsius. One calorie is equal to 4.2 kilojoules—a term used instead of calories in some countries.

Carbohydrates, classed as either simple (sugars) or complex (starches), are the main source of dietary energy. One gram of carbohydrates contains 4 calories. A healthy diet derives about 55% of calories from carbohydrates, with no more than 10% coming from sugars.

Saturated fat, derived from animal products and some tropical oils, has been found to raise blood cholesterol and should be limited to no more than one third of total fat calories.

Fiber in food aids elimination and helps prevent heart disease, intestinal disease and some forms of cancer. A healthy diet should include 20–35 grams of fiber daily.

A Note on Weights and Measures:
All recipes include customary U.S. and metric measurements. Metric conversions are based on a standard developed for these books and have been rounded off. Actual weights may vary. Unless otherwise stated, the recipes were designed for medium-sized fruits and vegetables.

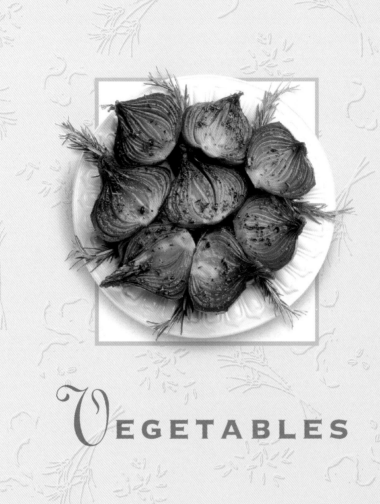

VEGETABLES

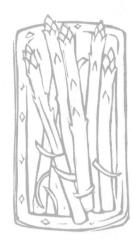

*I*f variety is the spice of life, then the recipes in this chapter will season meals for years to come. Vegetable side dishes present a delightful array of colors, textures and tastes that are pleasing to the eye, the palate and the healthy diet. Vegetables provide complex carbohydrates, fiber, very little fat and a spectrum of vitamins and minerals. Serving flavorful oven-roasted asparagus with sun-dried tomato vinaigrette, a snowy purée of cauliflower enriched with yogurt and cheese or sweet red onions baked whole will excite as much comment at meal time as any main dish or dessert. If selecting just one of these delicious alternatives is too difficult, make the wise choice of serving several side dishes to make up the entire meal. Because the highest nutritional content is found in fresh produce, these recipes are geared to combining seasonal vegetables. Every season offers fresh specialties, and many vegetables are available year round, meaning that the garden can always offer something good for the dining table.

The distinct flavors of this dish make it a great companion to grilled sausages or to whole fish baked with herbs. Sweet bell peppers, an excellent source of vitamin C, are available in an assortment of colors.

Tricolored Pepper Sauté

Serves 6

1 tablespoon olive oil
1 green bell pepper (capsicum), seeded, deribbed and cut into strips
1 red bell pepper (capsicum), seeded, deribbed and cut into strips
1 yellow bell pepper (capsicum), seeded, deribbed and cut into strips

1 small shallot, peeled and finely chopped
2 tablespoons dry white wine
1 teaspoon finely chopped fresh marjoram or ½ teaspoon dried marjoram
¼ teaspoon salt
⅛ teaspoon white pepper
2 teaspoons finely chopped fresh chives

1. In a sauté or frying pan over medium heat, warm the olive oil. Add the green, red and yellow bell peppers and sauté, stirring, until they just begin to soften, 2–3 minutes.
2. Add the shallot, wine, marjoram, salt and pepper. Reduce the heat slightly and simmer, uncovered, until the peppers are just tender, 3–4 minutes, stirring once halfway through. Remove from the heat and stir in the chives.
3. To serve, mound in a serving bowl.

Nutritional Analysis Per Serving:

CALORIES 34
(KILOJOULES 144)
PROTEIN 0 G
CARBOHYDRATES 3 G
TOTAL FAT 2 G
SATURATED FAT 0 G
CHOLESTEROL 0 MG
SODIUM 91 MG
DIETARY FIBER 1 G

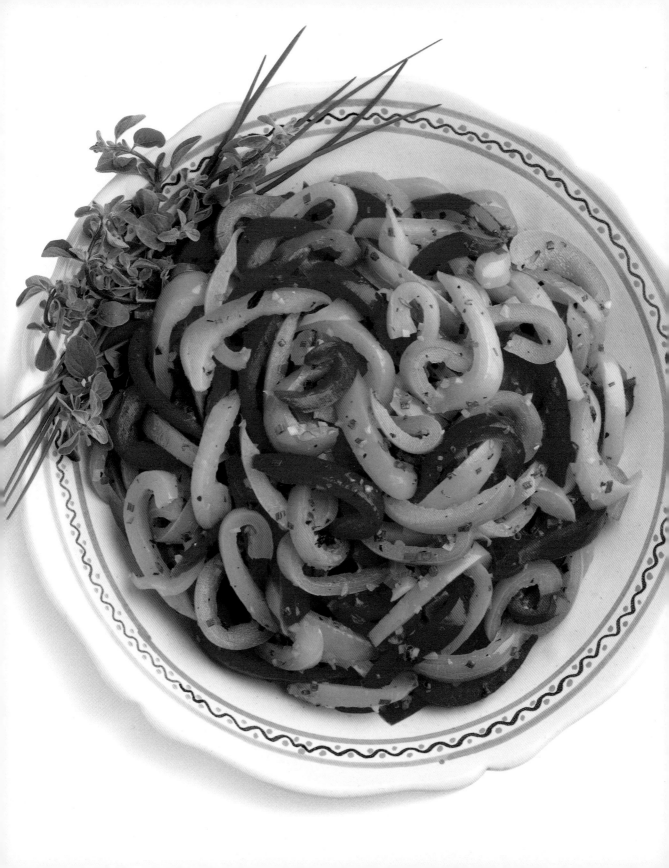

Double or triple this recipe to use as a barbecue party appetizer. Soak wooden or bamboo skewers in water to cover for 30 minutes to prevent burning. Tarragon vinegar imparts an almost sweet element to the marinade; different herbs will alter the flavor somewhat.

Grilled Mushrooms

Serves 4

2 tablespoons olive oil

2 teaspoons tarragon vinegar

½ teaspoon finely chopped
   fresh thyme or ¼ teaspoon
   dried thyme

1 teaspoon minced fresh basil

1 small shallot, peeled and minced

¼ teaspoon salt

⅛ teaspoon freshly ground pepper

1 lb (500 g) fresh button
   mushrooms, halved

1. Prepare a fire in a charcoal grill or preheat a broiler (griller). Away from the fire, coat the grill rack with nonstick cooking spray.

2. In a bowl, whisk together the olive oil, tarragon vinegar, thyme, basil, shallot, salt and pepper until well blended.

3. When the fire or broiler is ready, add the mushrooms to the olive oil mixture and toss gently but thoroughly to evenly coat with the marinade. Immediately begin to thread the mushrooms onto the skewers, running the skewer through the cut side of the mushrooms.

4. Place the skewers on the grill rack or on a broiler pan and grill or broil, turning to expose all sides to the heat, until the mushrooms are tender and golden, about 3 minutes on each side.

5. To serve, place the skewers on a serving dish.

*Nutritional Analysis
Per Serving:*

Calories 90

(Kilojoules 379)

Protein 2 g

Carbohydrates 6 g

Total Fat 7 g

Saturated Fat 1 g

Cholesterol 0 mg

Sodium 140 mg

Dietary Fiber 1 g

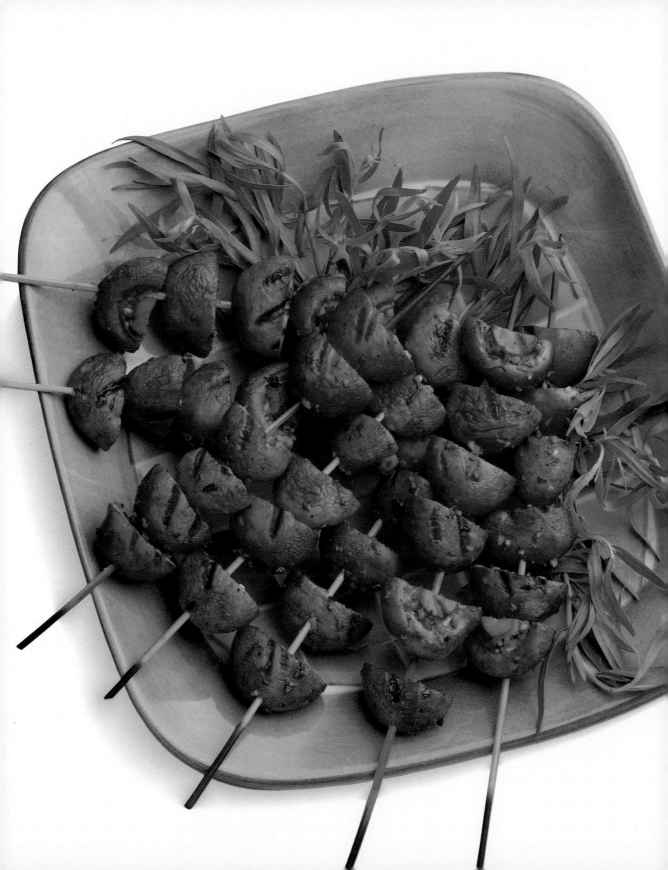

The honey in this recipe brings out the unexpectedly sweet flavor of parsnips. Select medium-sized parsnips and carrots for this dish, as larger vegetables may be tough. Add both the chive leaves and the edible purple flowers, if available, for an interesting presentation.

Glazed Carrots & Parsnips

Serves 4

2 tablespoons olive oil

3 carrots, peeled, halved lengthwise and cut into ¾-inch (2-cm) chunks

2 parsnips, peeled, quartered and cut into ¾-inch (2-cm) chunks

¼ cup (2 fl oz/60 ml) Chicken Stock *(recipe on page 127)* or water

1 tablespoon honey

¼ teaspoon salt

⅛ teaspoon coarsely cracked pepper

1 tablespoon finely chopped fresh chives

1. In a sauté or frying pan over medium heat, warm the olive oil. Add the carrots and parsnips and sauté, stirring occasionally, until just beginning to brown, 3–5 minutes.

2. Add the Chicken Stock or water, honey, salt and pepper and stir to mix well. Reduce the heat to low, cover and cook, stirring occasionally, until a glaze forms and the vegetables are just tender when pierced with a knife, 8–10 minutes.

3. Raise the heat to high and cook, stirring, until the glaze thickens enough to coat the vegetables, 2–3 minutes.

4. To serve, mound the vegetables in a serving bowl and sprinkle with the chives.

Nutritional Analysis Per Serving:

Calories 139

(Kilojoules 583)

Protein 1 g

Carbohydrates 19 g

Total Fat 7 g

Saturated Fat 1 g

Cholesterol 0 mg

Sodium 179 mg

Dietary Fiber 4 g

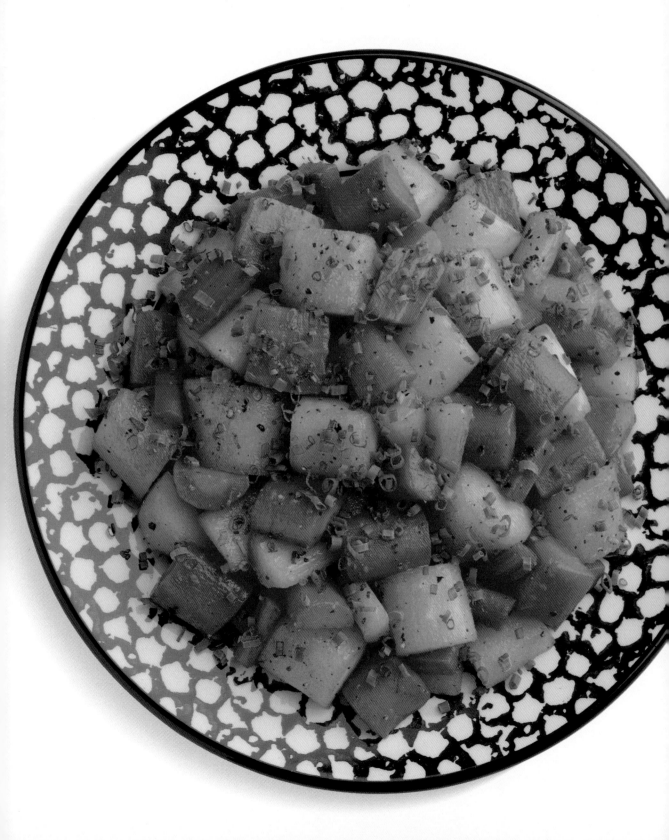

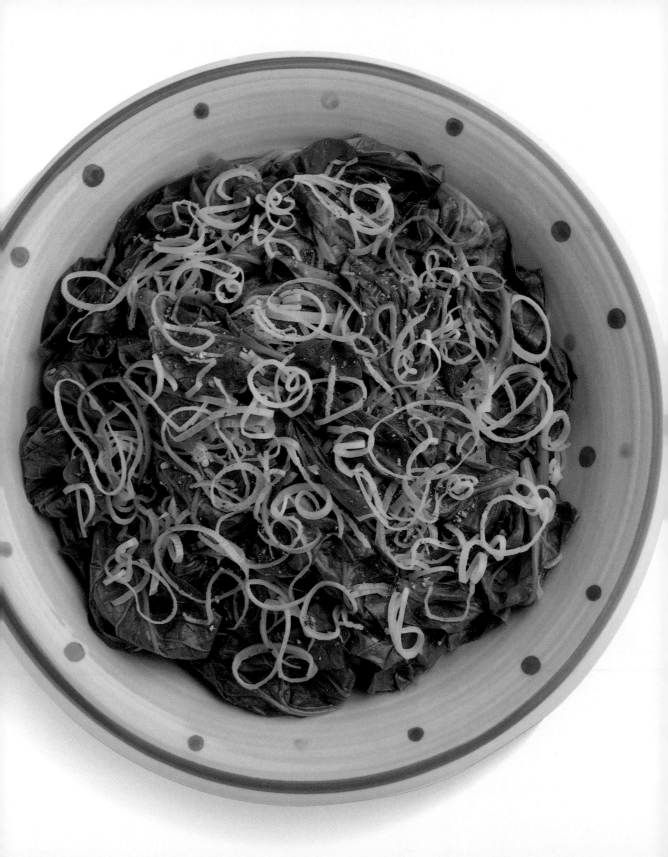

Spinach, a rich source of iron, gets a healthy Mediterranean-style cooking treatment when lightly steamed with leeks and lemon juice. Both vegetables require careful preparation (methods on pages 123 and 126). Try this dish with steamed fish.

Steamed Spinach & Leeks

Serves 4

1 tablespoon olive oil
2 leeks, green and white parts,
   thinly sliced
1 teaspoon fresh lemon juice
1 lb (500 g) fresh spinach leaves
   (about 3 bunches), tough
   stems removed

¼ teaspoon salt
⅛ teaspoon freshly ground
   pepper
1 teaspoon finely grated
   lemon zest
1 teaspoon sherry vinegar

1. In a heavy saucepan over medium heat, warm the olive oil. Add the leeks and sauté, stirring occasionally, until softened and translucent, 4–5 minutes.

2. Add the lemon juice and the spinach leaves, reduce the heat, cover and cook for 4 minutes without removing the lid. Uncover and toss to mix well.

3. Add the salt, pepper, lemon zest and sherry vinegar and cook, stirring, for 1 minute longer.

4. To serve, using a slotted spoon, transfer the vegetables to a serving dish.

Nutritional Analysis Per Serving:

**Calories 83
(Kilojoules 350)
Protein 3 g
Carbohydrates 11 g
Total Fat 4 g
Saturated Fat 1 g
Cholesterol 0 mg
Sodium 211 mg
Dietary Fiber 3 g**

This warm-weather side dish features a rainbow of vegetables. Feel free to substitute other fresh produce such as yellow squash for the butternut squash. Use long-handled tongs to turn the vegetables on the grill rack easily.

GRILLED VEGETABLES

Serves 6

2 tablespoons Mixed Herb Pesto *(recipe on page 127)*
2 tablespoons fresh lemon juice
⅓ cup (3 fl oz/80 ml) olive oil
2 red bell peppers (capsicums)
1 small butternut squash, 1 lb (500 g) peeled, seeded and cut lengthwise into strips

2 slender (Asian) eggplants (aubergines), halved lengthwise
2 zucchini (courgettes), halved lengthwise
3 large plum (Roma) tomatoes, 12 oz (375 g) total weight, halved lengthwise
¼ lb (125 g) button mushrooms, halved

Nutritional Analysis Per Serving:

CALORIES 195
(KILOJOULES 820)
PROTEIN 3 G
CARBOHYDRATES 17 G
TOTAL FAT 14 G
SATURATED FAT 2 G
CHOLESTEROL 1 MG
SODIUM 43 MG
DIETARY FIBER 2 G

1. Prepare a fire in a charcoal grill. Away from the fire, coat the grill rack with nonstick cooking spray.

2. To make the vinaigrette, in a small bowl, whisk together the Mixed Herb Pesto, lemon juice and olive oil until well blended.

3. Place the bell peppers on the grill rack and cook, turning occasionally, until the skins are blistered and slightly charred on all sides. Transfer the peppers to a brown paper bag, close the top tightly and let rest for 10 minutes. Remove the peppers from the bag and, using your fingers, peel off the charred skin. Halve the peppers and remove the seeds and ribs.

4. Place the butternut squash on the grill rack and cook, turning once, for 4–5 minutes on each side. Add the eggplant and zucchini slices and grill for 3 minutes on each side. Add the tomatoes and mushrooms and grill for 1–2 minutes on each side.

5. To serve, arrange the vegetables on a large platter. Drizzle with half of the vinaigrette (about 5 tablespoons). Pass the remaining vinaigrette.

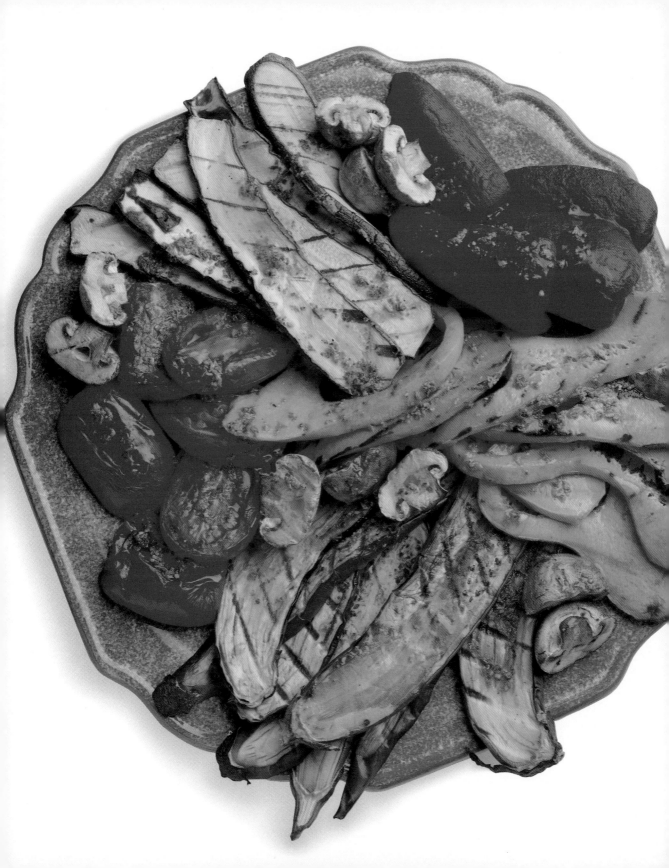

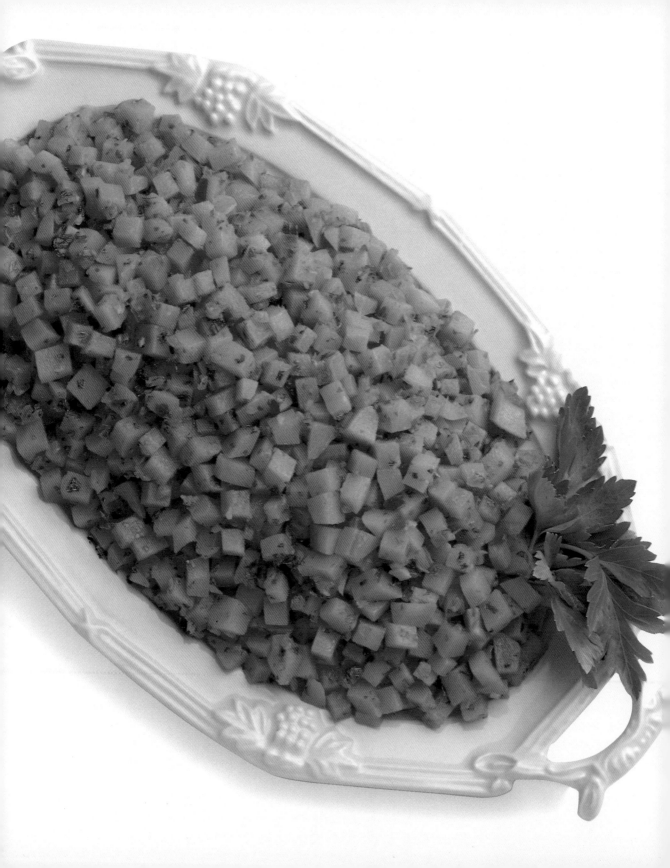

Try this cold-weather dish with a braised chicken or a roast turkey. Any sweet yellow onion, such as the Vidalia, Walla Walla or Maui varieties, may be substituted for the red onion to complement the sweetness of the squash.

Sautéed Winter Squash

Serves 6

2 tablespoons olive oil
½ red (Spanish) onion,
  finely chopped
2 teaspoons sherry vinegar
1 butternut squash, 2 lb (1 kg),
  peeled, seeded and diced
¼ teaspoon ground cumin

¾ cup (6 fl oz/180 ml) Chicken
  Stock *(recipe on page 127)*
  or water
½ teaspoon salt
¼ teaspoon white pepper
2 tablespoons finely chopped
  fresh parsley

1. In a large sauté or frying pan over medium heat, warm the olive oil. Add the onion and sauté, stirring occasionally, until softened and translucent, 5–6 minutes. Add the sherry vinegar and sauté until the vinegar is absorbed, 1–2 minutes longer.
2. Add the squash and continue to sauté over medium heat, stirring frequently, 3–5 minutes. Add the cumin, toss to coat and sauté for 1 minute longer. Add the Chicken Stock or water, cover and cook until the squash is tender when pierced with a fork, 5–7 minutes.
3. Remove from the heat and add the salt, pepper and parsley. Stir to mix well. If any liquid remains in the pan, place over high heat briefly to evaporate it.
4. To serve, spoon into a serving bowl.

Nutritional Analysis Per Serving:

**Calories 110
(Kilojoules 461)
Protein 2 g
Carbohydrates 17 g
Total Fat 5 g
Saturated Fat 1 g
Cholesterol 0 mg
Sodium 230 mg
Dietary Fiber 0 g**

Slow roasting caramelizes the natural sugars in vegetables, giving them a rich flavor and slight edge of sweetness—an especially pleasing effect on cabbage. You can roast this recipe at the same time you bake or roast a main dish.

Roasted Mixed Vegetables

Serves 6

3 carrots, peeled and cut
  into cubes
2 leeks, white part only,
  finely chopped
1 large eggplant (aubergine),
  1½ lb (750 g), cut into cubes
½ green cabbage, 1 lb (500 g),
  cored and sliced
8 garlic cloves, peeled and halved

3 tablespoons olive oil
1½ cups (12 fl oz/375 ml) Chicken
  Stock *(recipe on page 127)* or water
1 teaspoon finely chopped fresh thyme
  or ½ teaspoon dried thyme
1 tablespoon finely chopped fresh basil
3 tablespoons finely chopped fresh parsley
¼ teaspoon salt
¼ teaspoon freshly ground pepper

1. Preheat an oven to 400°F (200°C).
2. In a large roasting pan, combine the carrots, leeks, eggplant, cabbage, garlic, olive oil and Chicken Stock or water. Stir to mix well. Add the thyme, basil, 2 tablespoons of the parsley, the salt and pepper and stir to mix well. Be sure that all the vegetables are coated evenly.
3. Roast, turning the vegetables occasionally, until browned and caramelized, 45–60 minutes. You may need to raise the oven temperature to 425°F (220°C) for the last 15 minutes to caramelize the vegetables.
4. To serve, transfer to a serving bowl and garnish with the remaining 1 tablespoon parsley.

Nutritional Analysis Per Serving:

CALORIES 157
(KILOJOULES 661)
PROTEIN 4 G
CARBOHYDRATES 22 G
TOTAL FAT 7 G
SATURATED FAT 1 G
CHOLESTEROL 0 MG
SODIUM 208 MG
DIETARY FIBER 5 G

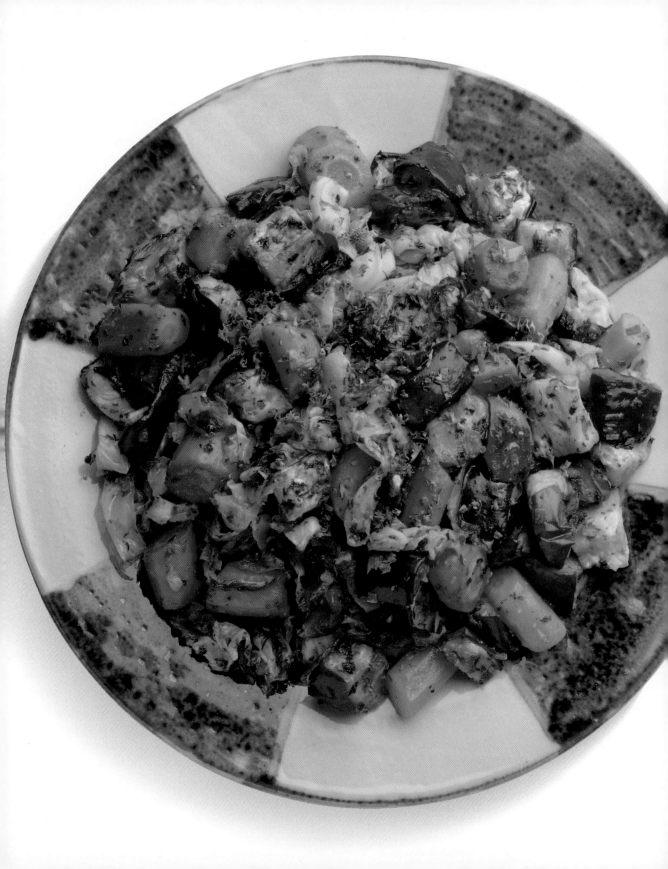

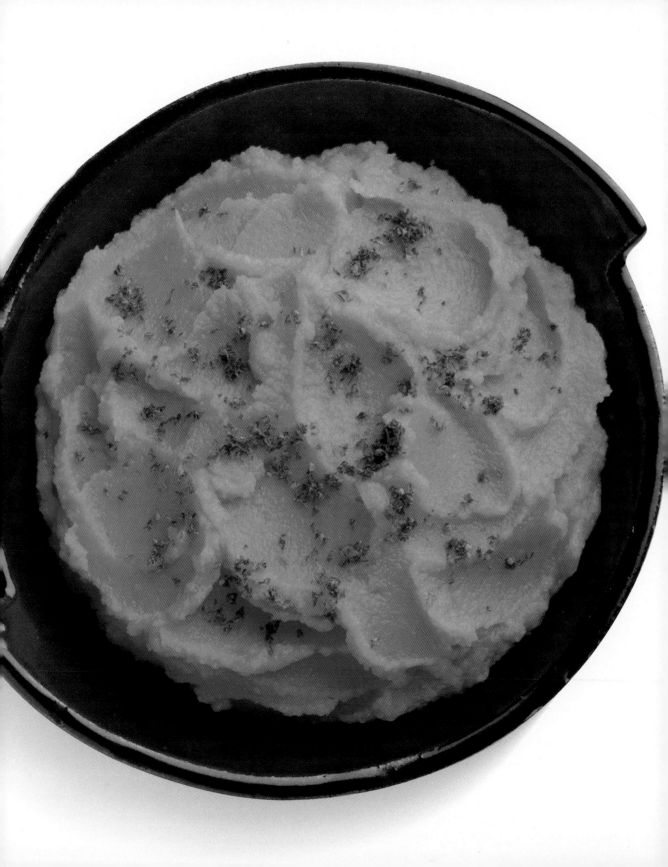

A little powdered ginger and white pepper provide a welcome balance to the sweetness of the squash and maple syrup in this winter side dish. Orange-fleshed squashes are especially high in vitamin A.

Butternut Squash Purée

Serves 4

1 butternut squash, 2 lb (1 kg), peeled, seeded and sliced
2 carrots, peeled, halved lengthwise and sliced
1 teaspoon ground ginger
1 tablespoon maple syrup

1½ tablespoons unsalted butter
1 tablespoon olive oil
¼ teaspoon salt
⅛ teaspoon white pepper
2 tablespoons finely chopped fresh parsley

1. Pour water to a depth of 1 inch (2.5 cm) in a steamer pan. Put the steamer rack in place and put the squash and carrot slices on the rack. Cover and bring the water to a boil. Steam over medium heat until tender when pierced with a fork, 15–20 minutes.
2. Transfer the squash and carrots to a food processor fitted with the metal blade. Add the ginger, maple syrup, butter, olive oil, salt and pepper and process until just puréed, scraping down the sides of the work bowl as necessary.
3. To serve, spoon into a serving bowl and garnish with the parsley.

Nutritional Analysis Per Serving:

CALORIES 185
(KILOJOULES 775)
PROTEIN 2 G
CARBOHYDRATES 30 G
TOTAL FAT 8 G
SATURATED FAT 3 G
CHOLESTEROL 12 MG
SODIUM 157 MG
DIETARY FIBER 1 G

If you can't find baby leeks measuring about ¾ inch (2 cm) in diameter, substitute larger leeks halved lengthwise. On all but the tiniest leeks, the outer-most layer can be tough, so take care to remove it before baking.

Baby Leek Gratin

Serves 4

2 tablespoons olive oil
10 baby leeks, 2¼ lb (1.1 kg) total
   weight, green and white parts
1 cup (8 fl oz/250 ml) Chicken
   Stock *(recipe on page 127)* or water
½ cup (2 oz/60 g) fine dried
   bread crumbs
2 tablespoons finely chopped
   fresh parsley
1 shallot, peeled and minced
2 teaspoons Dijon-style mustard
2 teaspoons olive oil

1. Preheat an oven to 350°F (180°C).
2. In an ovenproof frying pan large enough to hold the leeks in a single layer, over medium heat, warm the 2 tablespoons olive oil. Add the leeks and roll them to coat on all sides. Cook, uncovered, turning occasionally, until the leeks have just started to turn golden, 5–7 minutes.
3. Add the Chicken Stock or water and bring to a boil. Cover loosely with aluminum foil, then place the pan in the oven. Bake until the root ends of the leeks are tender when pierced with a knife, 10–15 minutes.
4. Coat a flameproof baking dish that can go directly to the table with nonstick cooking spray. Using a slotted spatula, transfer the leeks to the prepared dish.
5. Preheat a broiler (griller).
6. To make the topping, in a small bowl, stir together the bread crumbs, parsley, shallot, mustard and the 2 teaspoons olive oil. Sprinkle the mixture evenly over the leeks. Broil (grill) until browned and crisp, 2–3 minutes. Watch carefully that the bread crumbs do not burn.
7. Serve immediately from the baking dish.

*Nutritional Analysis
Per Serving:*

**Calories 304
(Kilojoules 1,277)
Protein 6 g
Carbohydrates 48 g
Total Fat 11 g
Saturated Fat 2 g
Cholesterol 0 mg
Sodium 330 mg
Dietary Fiber 4 g**

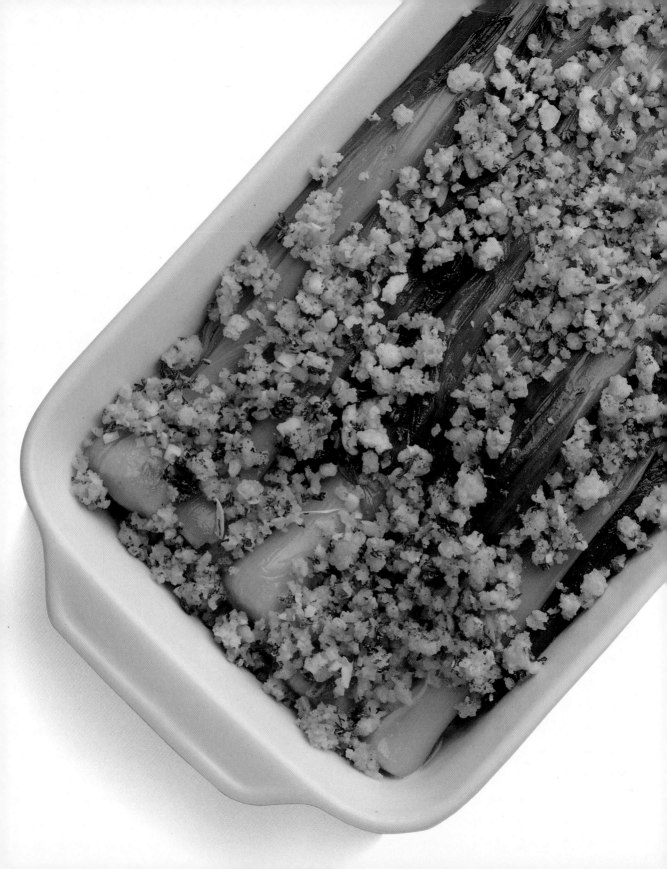

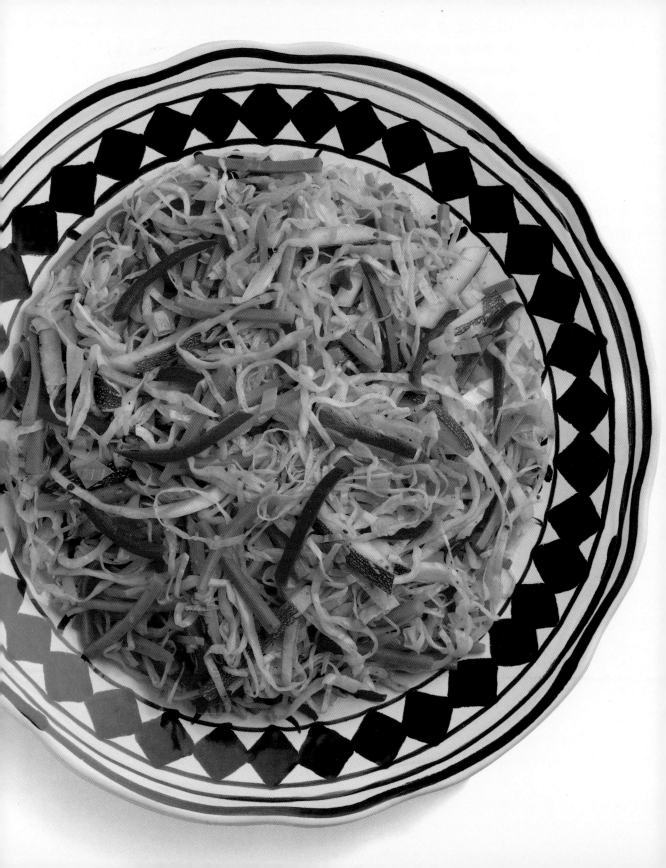

Quick cooking preserves much of cabbage's crunchy texture—as well as its nutrients. The spicy but not too hot flavor comes from a combination of curry powder and chili paste, both available in Asian food stores.

SPICY CABBAGE SAUTÉ

Serves 4

3 tablespoons olive oil
1 small leek, white part only,
   finely chopped
2 carrots, peeled and cut into strips
½ red bell pepper (capsicum),
   seeded, deribbed and cut
   into strips
1 zucchini (courgette), halved
   lengthwise and cut into strips

½ small green cabbage, ¾ lb (375 g),
   cored and finely shredded
1 teaspoon chili paste with garlic
½ teaspoon curry powder
¼ cup (2 fl oz/60 ml) water or
   Chicken Stock *(recipe on page 127)*
¼ teaspoon salt
⅛ teaspoon freshly ground pepper

1. In a sauté or deep frying pan over medium-high heat, warm the olive oil. Add the leek and sauté, stirring, until slightly softened, 3–4 minutes. Add the carrots, bell pepper and zucchini and sauté, stirring, until just tender, 3–4 minutes. Add the cabbage and toss to mix well. Cook, covered, until wilted, about 3 minutes longer.
2. Add the chili paste, curry powder, water or Chicken Stock, salt and pepper. Stir to mix well. Cover and cook for about 1 minute longer.
3. To serve, transfer to a serving bowl.

*Nutritional Analysis
Per Serving:*

**CALORIES 147
(KILOJOULES 618)
PROTEIN 2 G
CARBOHYDRATES 13 G
TOTAL FAT 11 G
SATURATED FAT 1 G
CHOLESTEROL 0 MG
SODIUM 174 MG
DIETARY FIBER 4 G**

These herb-flecked onions look especially pretty on a buffet table.
Also try cooking them outdoors by wrapping each onion in aluminum foil and
burying them in the hot coals of a barbecue for about 2 hours.

Baked Sweet Red Onions

Serves 8

4 red (Spanish) onions, halved
   from root to stem end with
   skin left intact
1½ tablespoons olive oil
¼ cup (2 fl oz/60 ml) Chicken
   Stock *(recipe on page 127)* or
   water
1 teaspoon balsamic vinegar

1 teaspoon sugar
1 teaspoon finely chopped fresh
   rosemary or ½ teaspoon dried
   rosemary
1 teaspoon finely chopped fresh thyme
   or ½ teaspoon dried thyme
½ teaspoon salt
¼ teaspoon freshly ground pepper

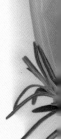

1. Preheat an oven to 350°F (180°C). Select a baking dish
in which the onion halves will fit in a single layer. Line it
with a piece of aluminum foil long enough to extend beyond
the ends and fold over to meet in the center. Lightly coat
the foil with nonstick cooking spray.

2. Place the onions, cut sides up, in the dish. Drizzle the
olive oil, Chicken Stock or water and balsamic vinegar
evenly over the onions. Sprinkle with the sugar, rosemary,
thyme, salt and pepper. Bring the ends of the foil together
to meet in the center, covering the onions loosely.

3. Bake for 1 hour. Fold back the foil to expose the onions.
Continue to bake until the onions are very tender when
pierced with a fork, 30–45 minutes longer.

4. To serve, transfer to a serving platter.

*Nutritional Analysis
Per Serving:*

**Calories 73
(Kilojoules 307)
Protein 2 g
Carbohydrates 11 g
Total Fat 3 g
Saturated Fat 0 g
Cholesterol 0 mg
Sodium 159 mg
Dietary Fiber 2 g**

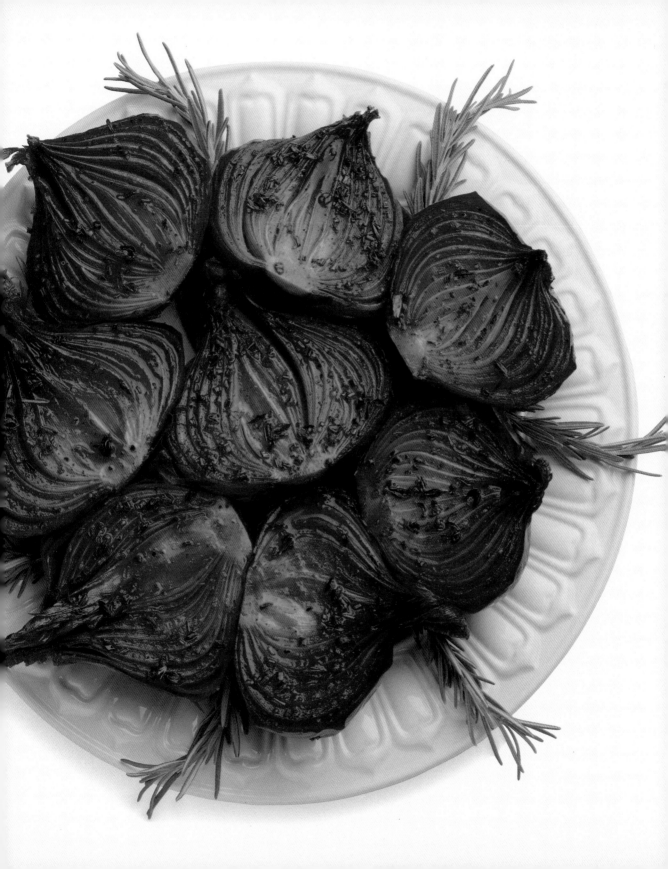

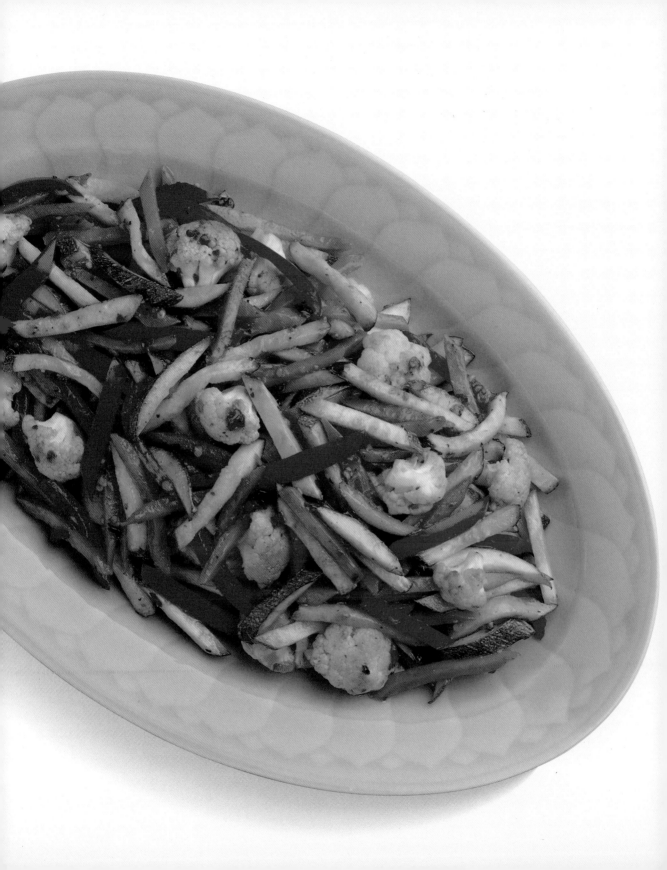

Because this dish goes together very quickly, assemble all the ingredients in small bowls near the stove before you begin cooking. The black bean sauce, available in Asian food stores and well-stocked groceries, has a slightly salty flavor.

Stir-Fried Vegetables in Black Bean Sauce

Serves 4

1 tablespoon vegetable oil

2 carrots, peeled and cut into strips

1 cup (3 oz/90 g) cauliflower florets (from ½ medium head)

1 garlic clove, peeled and minced

1 teaspoon peeled and minced fresh ginger

1 lb (500 g) zucchini (courgettes), halved lengthwise and cut into strips

1 red bell pepper (capsicum), seeded, deribbed and cut into strips

2 teaspoons black bean sauce

2 teaspoons low sodium soy sauce

1 tablespoon dry sherry

2 teaspoons cornstarch dissolved in 2 tablespoons water or Chicken Stock *(recipe on page 127)*

1. In a large, deep nonstick frying pan or a wok over medium-high heat, warm the vegetable oil, swirling it around in the pan. When it is hot, add the carrots, cauliflower, garlic and ginger and cook, tossing occasionally, until coated with the oil and lightly glazed, about 1½ minutes.

2. Add the zucchini, bell pepper and bean sauce and continue to cook, stirring constantly, until all the vegetables are beginning to soften, 3–4 minutes.

3. Add the soy sauce, sherry and cornstarch mixture, stir to mix well and cook, stirring, until slightly thickened, 1 minute longer.

4. To serve, transfer to a serving bowl.

Nutritional Analysis Per Serving:

Calories 89
(Kilojoules 372)
Protein 3 g
Carbohydrates 12 g
Total Fat 4 g
Saturated Fat 0 g
Cholesterol 0 mg
Sodium 240 mg
Dietary Fiber 3 g

A combination of nonfat yogurt, ricotta and Cheddar cheeses provides all the home-style satisfaction of old-fashioned cauliflower and cheese, while having only a fraction of the fat. This dish goes particularly well with pork.

Cauliflower Purée

Serves 4

4½ cups (13½ oz/425 g) cauliflower florets (from 1 large head)
3 tablespoons nonfat plain yogurt or nonfat sour cream
½ cup (4 oz/125 g) lowfat ricotta cheese
⅓ cup (1½ oz/45 g) grated Cheddar cheese
½ teaspoon Dijon-style mustard
½ teaspoon salt
⅛ teaspoon white pepper
2 tablespoons finely chopped fresh chives

1. Pour water to a depth of 1 inch (2.5 cm) in a steamer pan. Put the steamer rack in place and the cauliflower on the rack. Cover and bring the water to a boil. Steam over medium heat until tender when pierced with a fork, 12–15 minutes.

2. Transfer the cauliflower to a food processor fitted with the metal blade. Purée until smooth, scraping down the sides of the work bowl as necessary. Add the yogurt or sour cream, ricotta and Cheddar cheeses, mustard, salt and pepper and process just until blended.

3. To serve, mound in a serving bowl and garnish with the chives.

Nutritional Analysis Per Serving:

CALORIES 108
(KILOJOULES 454)
PROTEIN 9 G
CARBOHYDRATES 7 G
TOTAL FAT 6 G
SATURATED FAT 3 G
CHOLESTEROL 16 MG
SODIUM 416 MG
DIETARY FIBER 2 G

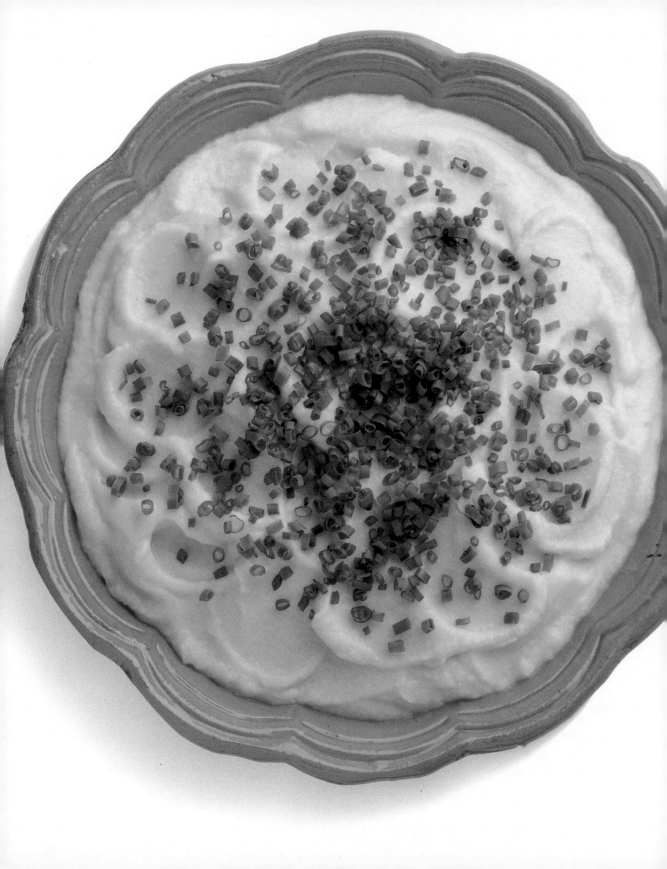

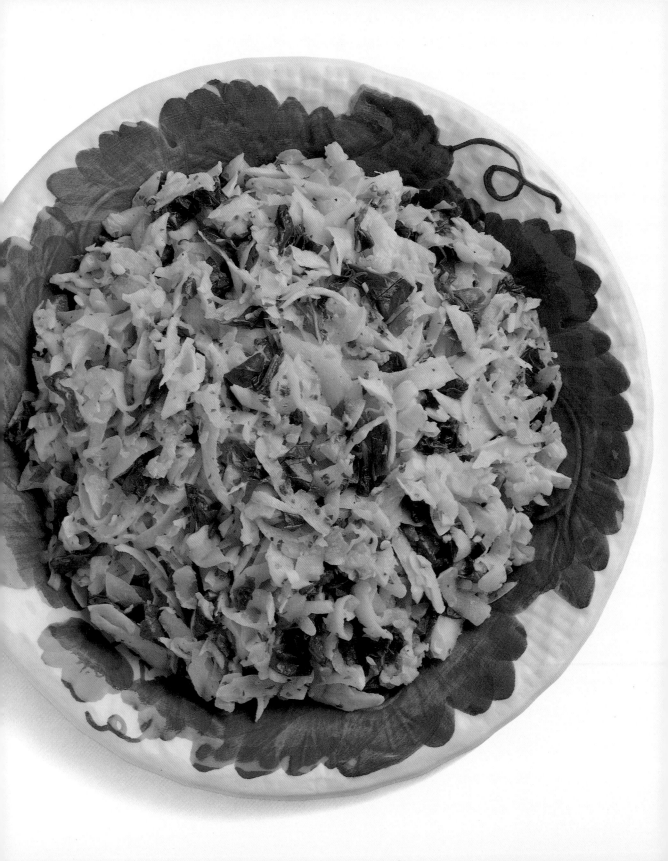

Mild summer squash gets a lift from peppery arugula leaves and tangy lemon. Arugula tastes similar to watercress. Its flavor is best when the leaves are young and tender. The resulting side dish goes beautifully with grilled fish.

Yellow Squash & Arugula Medley

Serves 4

4 yellow summer squashes, about
    1 lb (500 g) total weight,
    coarsely grated
2 tablespoons olive oil
1 cup (1 oz/30 g) coarsely
    chopped arugula (rocket)
1 shallot, peeled and finely
    chopped

1 garlic clove, peeled and minced
1 teaspoon grated lemon zest
1 tablespoon fresh lemon juice
1 tablespoon finely chopped
    fresh parsley
¼ teaspoon salt
⅛ teaspoon freshly ground pepper

1. Place the squashes in a clean kitchen towel and wring out all excess moisture.
2. In a sauté or frying pan over medium heat, warm the olive oil. Add the squash and sauté, stirring gently, for 2 minutes.
3. Add the arugula and shallot and continue to sauté, stirring gently, until the arugula has just begun to wilt and the shallot is softened, 1–2 minutes. Add the garlic, lemon zest and juice, parsley, salt and pepper. Stir to mix well. Sauté 1 minute longer.
4. To serve, transfer to a serving bowl.

Nutritional Analysis Per Serving:

**CALORIES 88
(KILOJOULES 368)
PROTEIN 2 G
CARBOHYDRATES 6 G
TOTAL FAT 7 G
SATURATED FAT 1 G
CHOLESTEROL 0 MG
SODIUM 141 MG
DIETARY FIBER 2 G**

Subtle touches of two ingredients with strong personalities—fresh mint and jalapeño pepper—give a wonderful complexity to this simple summertime dish. Take care to wash your hands and utensils well after handling the chili.

SPICY SUMMER SAUTÉ

Serves 6

2 tablespoons olive oil
2 zucchini (courgettes), sliced
1 eggplant (aubergine), peeled and sliced
1 red bell pepper (capsicum), seeded, deribbed and cut into strips
1 garlic clove, peeled and minced

2 tablespoons finely chopped fresh mint
½ teaspoon finely chopped fresh jalapeño pepper
¼ cup (2 fl oz/60 ml) Chicken Stock *(recipe on page 127)* or water
¼ teaspoon salt
⅛ teaspoon freshly ground pepper

1. In a sauté or large frying pan over medium-high heat, warm the olive oil. Add the zucchini, eggplant and bell pepper and sauté, tossing frequently, until lightly browned, 5–6 minutes.
2. Reduce the heat to medium and add the garlic, 1 tablespoon of the mint and the jalapeño. Continue to sauté for 1 minute longer. Turn the heat to medium-high and add the Chicken Stock or water. Continue to sauté, stirring occasionally, until the liquid has almost evaporated and the vegetables are tender, about 2 minutes longer.
3. Add the salt and pepper and stir to mix well. Add the remaining 1 tablespoon mint and mix well.
4. To serve, transfer to a large dish.

Nutritional Analysis Per Serving:

CALORIES 76
(KILOJOULES 318)
PROTEIN 2 G
CARBOHYDRATES 8 G
TOTAL FAT 5 G
SATURATED FAT 1 G
CHOLESTEROL 0 MG
SODIUM 109 MG
DIETARY FIBER 2 G

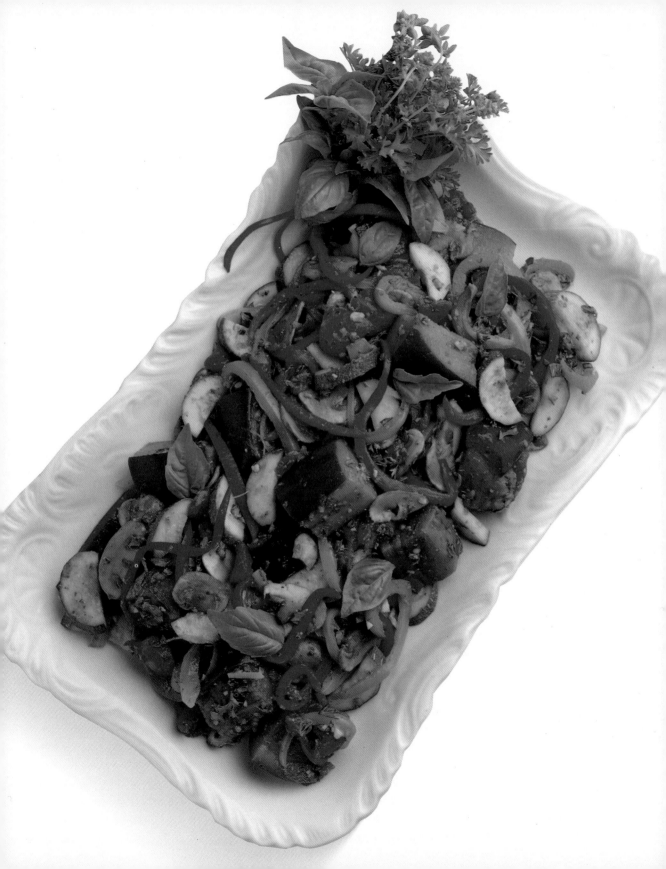

This flavorful dressing uses less oil than conventional vinaigrettes. Roasting complements the crisp texture of asparagus, which is rich in vitamin A and potassium. Sun-dried tomatoes retain the vitamins and minerals of fresh tomatoes, just in more concentrated form.

Asparagus with Sun-Dried Tomato Vinaigrette

Serves 6

1½ lb (750 g) thin asparagus, trimmed and bottom 2 inches (5 cm) peeled
¼ cup (2 fl oz/60 ml) Chicken Stock *(recipe on page 127)* or water
1 tablespoon finely chopped fresh parsley

Sun-Dried Tomato Vinaigrette

¼ cup (1½ oz/45 g) sun-dried tomatoes, dry-packed, soaked in very hot water for 30 minutes, drained and blotted dry
1 garlic clove, peeled and coarsely chopped
1 shallot, peeled and coarsely chopped
2 tablespoons red wine vinegar
2 teaspoons fresh lemon juice
¼ teaspoon salt
⅛ teaspoon freshly ground pepper
1 tablespoon finely chopped fresh basil
⅓ cup (3 fl oz/80 ml) olive oil

Nutritional Analysis Per Serving:

CALORIES 131
(KILOJOULES 550)
PROTEIN 2 G
CARBOHYDRATES 5 G
TOTAL FAT 12 G
SATURATED FAT 2 G
CHOLESTEROL 0 MG
SODIUM 108 MG
DIETARY FIBER 1 G

1. Preheat an oven to 350°F (180°C).

2. In a roasting pan, combine the asparagus and Chicken Stock or water. Roast until just tender when pierced with a fork, 10–15 minutes. The timing will depend upon the size of the asparagus. Remove from the oven and drain well. Cover and refrigerate until well chilled, about 3 hours.

3. Prepare the Sun-Dried Tomato Vinaigrette (see below).

4. To serve, arrange the asparagus on a serving platter. Top with half of the Sun-Dried Tomato Vinaigrette (about 5 tablespoons). Sprinkle with the reserved sun-dried tomato strips and the parsley. Pass the remaining vinaigrette.

Sun-Dried Tomato Vinaigrette

1. Cut the sun-dried tomatoes into thin strips, reserving a few strips for garnishing.

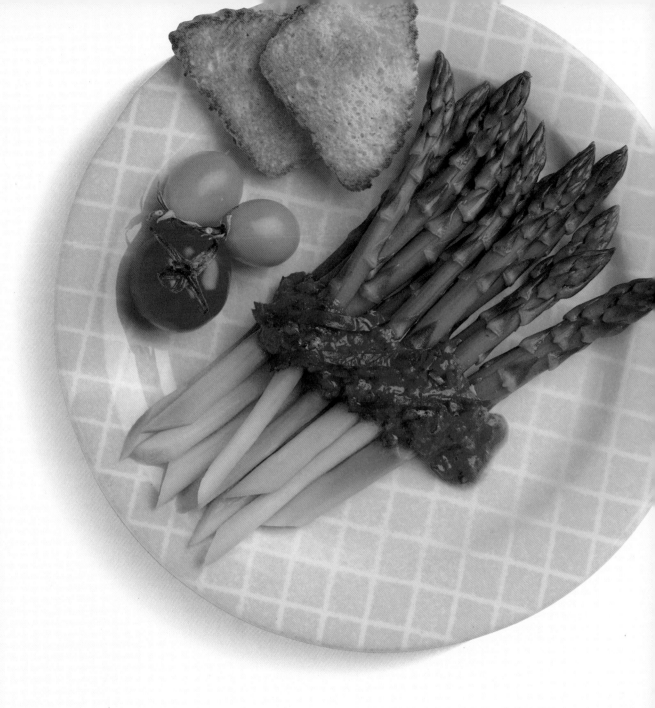

2. In a food processor fitted with the metal blade, combine the garlic, shallot and sun-dried tomatoes. Process until minced. Add the red wine vinegar, lemon juice, salt, pepper and basil. Process until combined. With the motor running, slowly add the olive oil in a thin, steady stream.

Often overlooked, the yellow-fleshed rutabaga is paired here with its smaller cousin, the crisp, white-fleshed turnip. This unexpected side dish combination provides a good source of vitamins A and C and iron.

Turnip & Rutabaga Purée

Serves 6

1¼ lb (625 g) white turnips, peeled and cut into cubes
1¼ lb (625 g) rutabagas (swedes), peeled and cut into cubes
2 garlic cloves, peeled and minced
2 tablespoons olive oil
½ teaspoon ground allspice
¼ teaspoon ground nutmeg
¼ teaspoon salt
¼ teaspoon freshly ground pepper
3 tablespoons lowfat buttermilk
3 fresh parsley sprigs

1. Fill a large saucepan three-fourths full of water, add the turnips and rutabagas and place over medium-high heat. Bring to a boil, cover partially and cook until tender, 15–17 minutes. Drain well.

2. In a food processor fitted with the metal blade, combine the turnips, rutabagas and garlic. Purée until smooth. Add the olive oil, allspice, nutmeg, salt, pepper and buttermilk and process to mix well, scraping down the sides of the work bowl as necessary.

3. To serve, transfer to a serving bowl and garnish with the parsley sprigs.

Nutritional Analysis Per Serving:

Calories 95
(Kilojoules 400)
Protein 2 g
Carbohydrates 12 g
Total Fat 5 g
Saturated Fat 1 g
Cholesterol 0 mg
Sodium 166 mg
Dietary Fiber 3 g

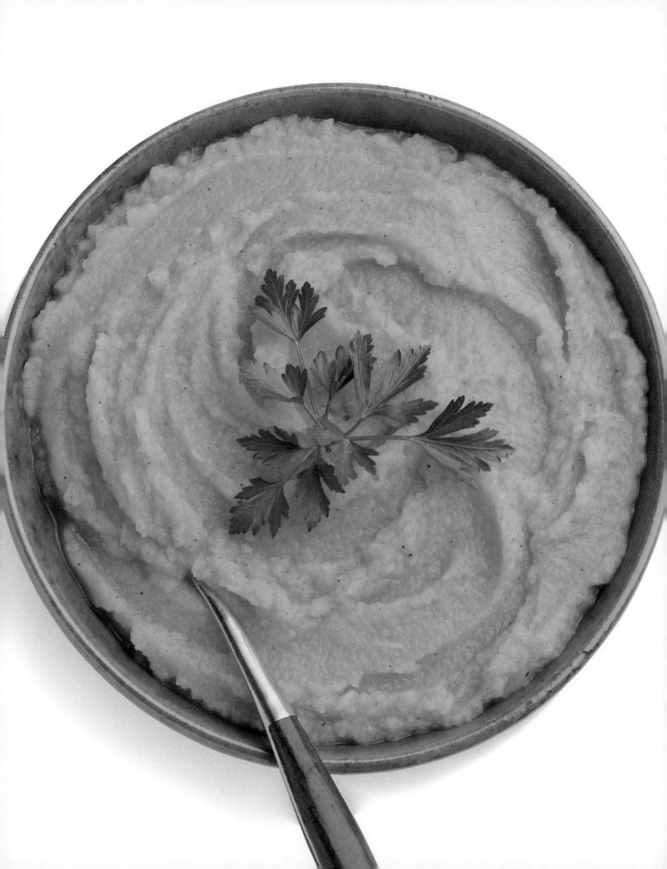

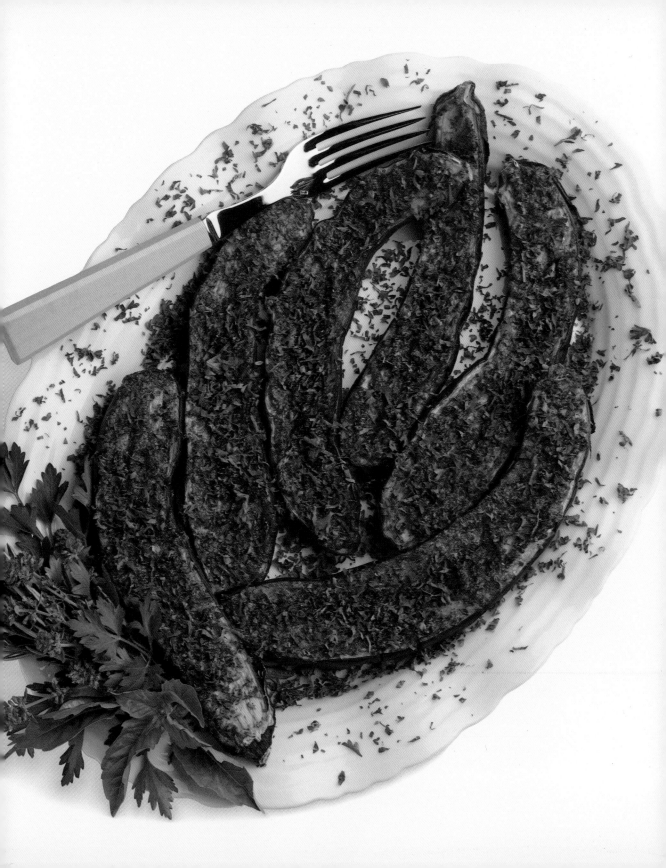

Mixed Herb Pesto highlights eggplant's mild flavor and forms a crisp crust during baking. For the best results, seek out the slender variety known as Japanese or Asian eggplants. Parsley is well used here, providing a crisp texture and vitamin C.

Baked Eggplant

Serves 6

3 slender (Asian) eggplants
  (aubergines), halved lengthwise
¼ cup (2 fl oz/60 ml) Mixed Herb
  Pesto *(recipe on page 127)*
3 tablespoons finely chopped fresh parsley

1. Preheat an oven to 350°F (180°C).
2. Place the eggplants, cut sides up, in a roasting pan. Prick the cut sides with a sharp knife and spread with an equal amount of the Mixed Herb Pesto.
3. Bake until the eggplants are tender and the tops are well browned, 40–45 minutes.
4. To serve, arrange on a warmed platter and sprinkle with the parsley.

Nutritional Analysis Per Serving:

CALORIES 55
(KILOJOULES 230)
PROTEIN 2 G
CARBOHYDRATES 5 G
TOTAL FAT 4 G
SATURATED FAT 1 G
CHOLESTEROL 2 MG
SODIUM 64 MG
DIETARY FIBER 1 G

Topped as they are with a garlicky sauté of tomatoes, onion, carrots and fresh herbs, the strands of this unusual winter squash really do resemble spaghetti—particularly if you present this side dish in a large, shallow pasta bowl.

Baked Spaghetti Squash

Serves 6

1 spaghetti squash, 2 lb (1 kg)
1 tablespoon olive oil
1 yellow onion, finely chopped
2 carrots, peeled and finely chopped
2 garlic cloves, peeled and minced
3 large plum (Roma) tomatoes,
  12 oz (375 g) total weight, peeled,
  seeded and coarsely chopped

1 tablespoon chopped fresh parsley
1 tablespoon finely chopped
  fresh basil
1 tablespoon finely chopped
  fresh chives
¼ teaspoon salt
⅛ teaspoon freshly ground pepper
½ cup (2 oz/60 g) crumbled feta
  cheese

1. Preheat an oven to 350°F (180°C).
2. Prick the squash all over with a fork and place on a rack in a roasting pan. Bake until tender when pierced with a fork, about 1 hour and 10 minutes, turning the squash over halfway through.
3. Meanwhile, in a frying pan over medium heat, warm the olive oil. Add the onion and carrots and cook, uncovered, until softened, 5–7 minutes. Add the garlic, tomatoes, parsley, basil, chives, salt and pepper and stir to mix well. Reduce the heat to low, cover partially and simmer for 10 minutes longer. Keep warm.
4. When the squash is ready, remove from the oven and halve horizontally. Scoop out the seeds and discard. Using a fork, scrape out the flesh from the rind. It should pull out in long, spaghetti-like strands.
5. Mound the squash in a large, shallow serving bowl. Spoon the warm vegetable mixture over the squash and toss gently to mix. Scatter the feta cheese over the top.

Nutritional Analysis Per Serving:

Calories 124
(Kilojoules 522)
Protein 4 g
Carbohydrates 16 g
Total Fat 6 g
Saturated Fat 2 g
Cholesterol 7 mg
Sodium 172 mg
Dietary Fiber 2 g

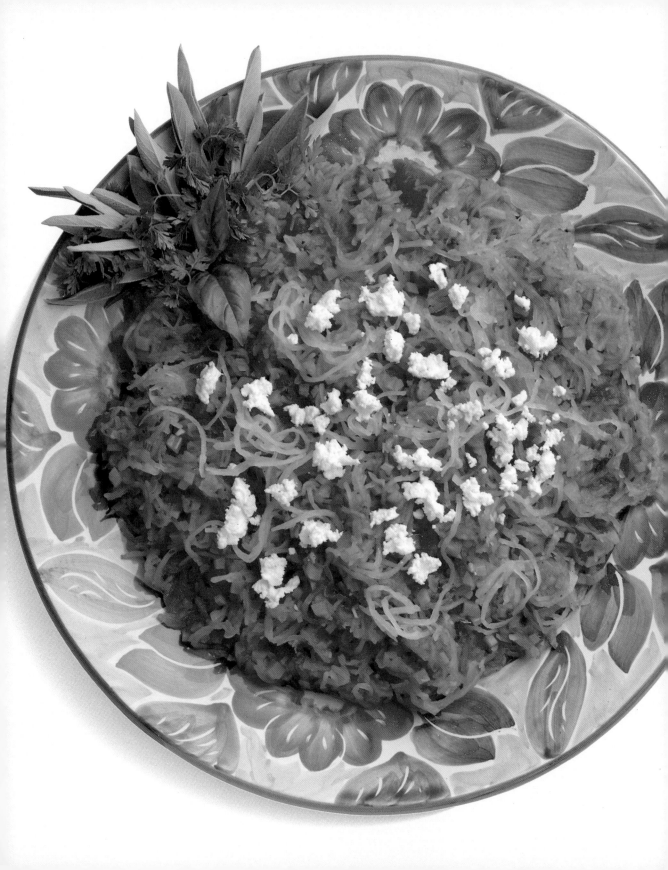

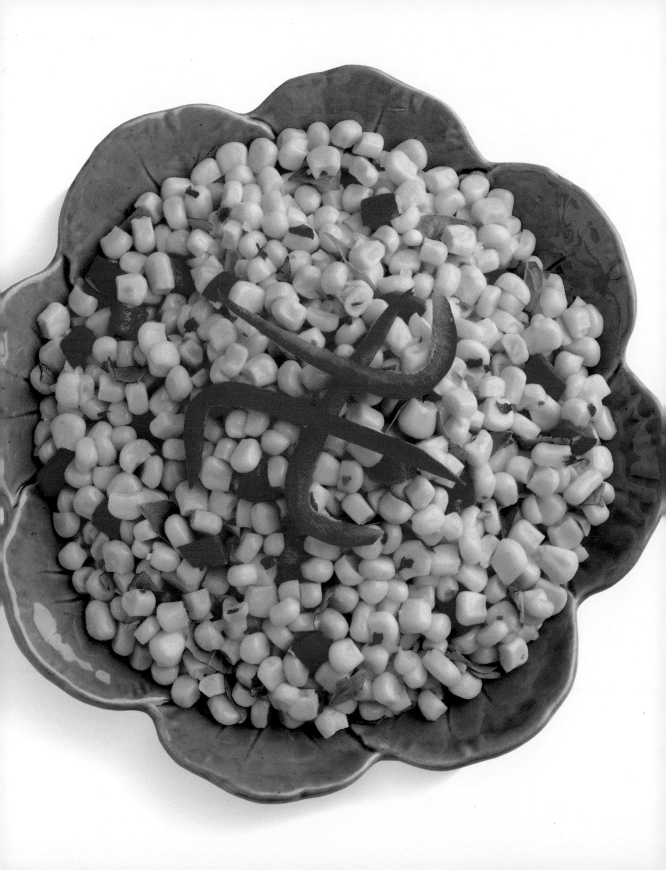

Try making this when fresh sweet corn is in season, as an accompaniment to grilled chicken or steak. About ⅛ teaspoon of hot chili oil may be substituted for the pepper flakes and either may be increased for spicier results.

Sautéed Corn & Red Pepper

Serves 4

1 tablespoon olive oil

2 tablespoons coarsely chopped red bell pepper (capsicum)

3 cups (18 oz/560 g) fresh or thawed frozen corn kernels (from 5–6 ears)

2 garlic cloves, peeled and minced

¼ teaspoon salt

⅛ teaspoon red pepper flakes, crushed

2 tablespoons chopped fresh basil

1. In a sauté or frying pan over medium heat, warm the olive oil. Add the bell pepper and sauté, stirring occasionally, until just tender, 2–3 minutes. Add the corn kernels and garlic and sauté, stirring, until the kernels begin to release their liquid, 1–2 minutes.

2. Add the salt and red pepper flakes and cook for 1 minute longer.

3. To serve, transfer to a serving bowl and stir in the basil.

Nutritional Analysis Per Serving:

**Calories 144
(Kilojoules 606)
Protein 4 g
Carbohydrates 25 g
Total Fat 5 g
Saturated Fat 1 g
Cholesterol 0 mg
Sodium 155 mg
Dietary Fiber 4 g**

This popular southern French medley of summer vegetables is usually sautéed with a large measure of olive oil. Here, baking in the oven delivers all the traditional flavor with far less fat.

Oven-Baked Ratatouille

Serves 6

1 eggplant (aubergine), cut into cubes

2 medium or 1 large yellow onion, thinly sliced

1 red bell pepper (capsicum), seeded, deribbed and thinly sliced

½ green bell pepper (capsicum), seeded, deribbed and thinly sliced

2 teaspoons finely chopped fresh thyme or 1 teaspoon dried thyme

3 tablespoons olive oil

¼ lb (125 g) button mushrooms, thinly sliced

1 garlic clove, peeled and minced

1½ cups (9 oz/280 g) crushed tomatoes

½ teaspoon salt

¼ teaspoon freshly ground pepper

2 zucchini (courgettes), halved lengthwise and thinly sliced

2 tablespoons finely chopped fresh parsley

2 tablespoons finely chopped fresh basil

¼ cup (2 fl oz/60 ml) Mixed Herb Pesto *(recipe on page 127)*

1. Preheat an oven to 425°F (220°C).
2. In a large roasting pan, combine the eggplant, onion, red and green bell peppers and thyme. Drizzle with the olive oil and toss to coat well. Bake until all the vegetables begin to soften, 20–25 minutes, stirring once about halfway through.
3. Add the mushrooms, garlic, tomatoes, salt and pepper. Toss to mix well. Return to the oven and bake until the tomatoes have started to break down, 10–15 minutes longer, stirring once about halfway through.
4. Add the zucchini, parsley and basil and toss to mix well. Return to the oven and bake until the zucchini is tender, 8–10 minutes longer.
5. To serve, using a slotted spoon, transfer the mixture to a heated serving dish. Discard the excess liquid. Add the Mixed Herb Pesto and stir to mix well.

Nutritional Analysis Per Serving:

CALORIES 173
(KILOJOULES 727)
PROTEIN 4 G
CARBOHYDRATES 18 G
TOTAL FAT 11 G
SATURATED FAT 2 G
CHOLESTEROL 2 MG
SODIUM 322 MG
DIETARY FIBER 3 G

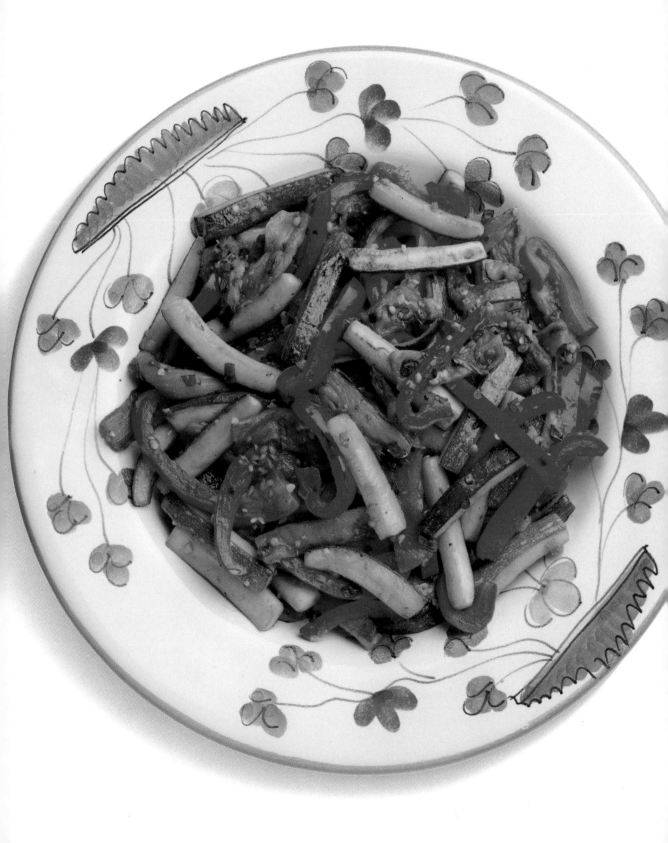

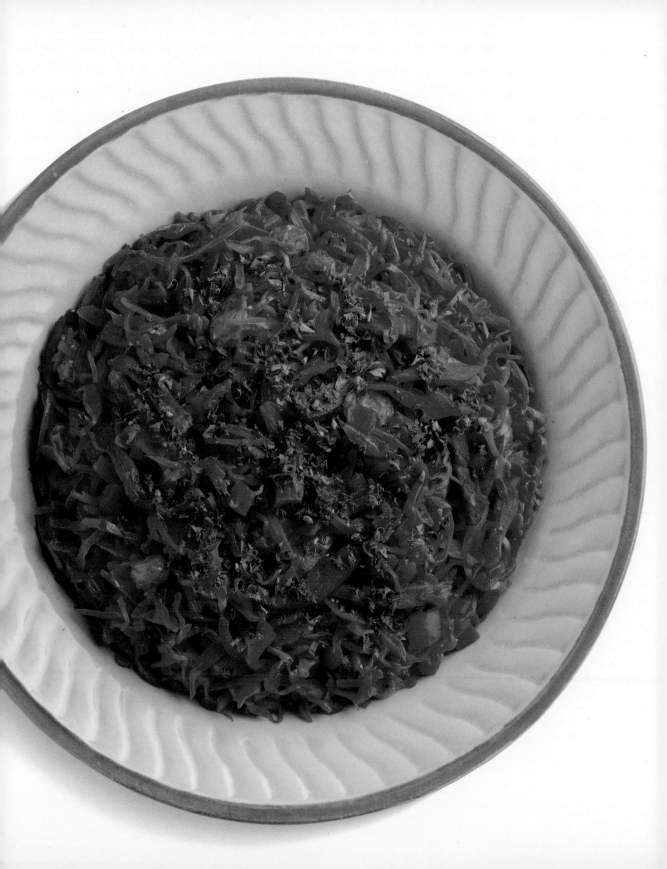

Savory and comforting, this luscious winter cabbage dish goes well with grilled chicken or turkey sausages. Although cooked for a long time, the cabbage retains a slightly crisp bite and lean Canadian bacon adds a hint of smoky flavor.

Braised Cabbage & Canadian Bacon

Serves 6

2 tablespoons olive oil

1 small yellow onion, finely chopped

1 small carrot, peeled and finely chopped

3 oz (90 g) Canadian bacon, cut into strips

1 red cabbage, about 2 lb (1 kg), cored and shredded

1 green apple, peeled, cored and coarsely chopped

¼ cup (1½ oz/45 g) golden raisins (sultanas)

1 cup (8 fl oz/250 ml) dry red wine

1 cup (8 fl oz/250 ml) Chicken Stock *(recipe on page 127)* or water

½ teaspoon salt

¼ teaspoon freshly ground pepper

½ teaspoon sugar

1 tablespoon finely chopped fresh parsley

1. In a heavy saucepan over medium heat, warm the olive oil. Add the onion, carrot and bacon and sauté, stirring, until the vegetables are softened, 5–6 minutes.

2. Add the cabbage, apple and raisins and continue to cook over medium heat, stirring occasionally, until the cabbage begins to soften, 5–6 minutes.

3. Add the wine, Chicken Stock or water, salt, pepper and sugar. Stir to mix well. Cover, reduce the heat to very low and simmer gently until very tender, 45–60 minutes.

4. To serve, using a slotted spoon, transfer the vegetables to a serving bowl and garnish with the parsley.

Nutritional Analysis Per Serving:

CALORIES 149
(KILOJOULES 626)
PROTEIN 6 G
CARBOHYDRATES 21 G
TOTAL FAT 6 G
SATURATED FAT 1 G
CHOLESTEROL 7 MG
SODIUM 456 MG
DIETARY FIBER 4 G

Snow peas, also known as Chinese pea pods, taste their best when crispy, so take care not to cook them too long. The mixed yellow and red bell pepper add a nice contrast of color, along with vitamin C.

Sautéed Peppers & Snow Peas

Serves 6

1½ tablespoons olive oil
1 red bell pepper (capsicum), seeded, deribbed and cut into strips
1 yellow bell pepper (capsicum), seeded, deribbed and cut into strips
¾ lb (375 g) snow peas (mangetouts), ends trimmed
¼ teaspoon salt
⅛ teaspoon freshly ground pepper
2 teaspoons finely chopped fresh chives

1. In a sauté or frying pan over medium heat, warm the olive oil. Add the red and yellow peppers and sauté, stirring, until just beginning to soften, 1–2 minutes.
2. Add the snow peas and sauté until the peas are just tender, 1–2 minutes longer. Add the salt and pepper and toss to mix well.
3. To serve, mound in a serving bowl and garnish with the chives.

Nutritional Analysis Per Serving:

Calories 60
(Kilojoules 253)
Protein 2 g
Carbohydrates 6 g
Total Fat 4 g
Saturated Fat 0 g
Cholesterol 0 mg
Sodium 93 mg
Dietary Fiber 2 g

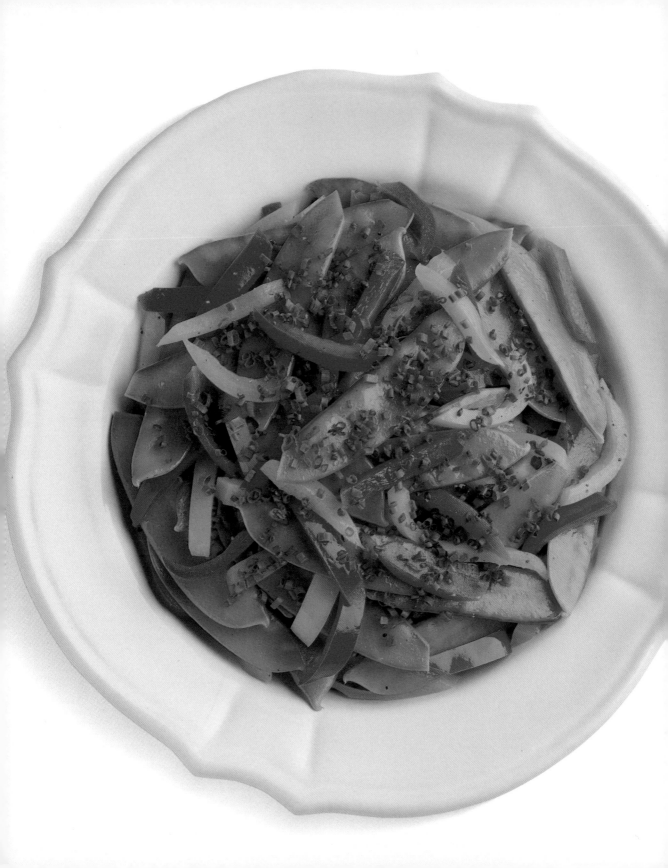

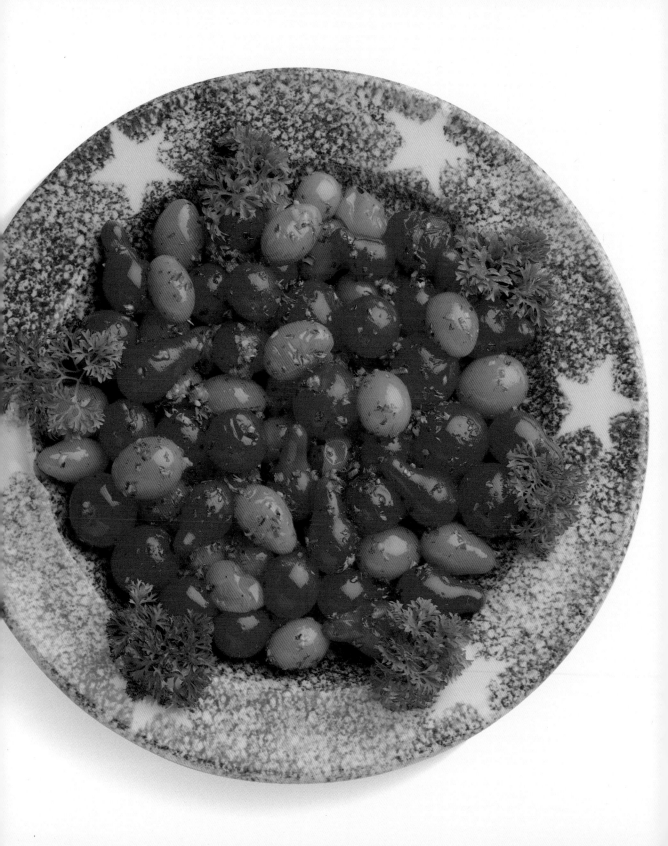

Baking in the oven intensifies the flavors of sweet, juicy cherry tomatoes, which gain a Mediterranean accent in this recipe thanks to shallots, garlic, thyme, parsley and a hint of olive oil. Both yellow and red tomatoes work well for this dish.

BAKED CHERRY TOMATOES

Serves 6

1 lb (500 g) cherry tomatoes,
  stems removed
1 shallot, peeled and finely chopped
1 garlic clove, peeled and minced
½ teaspoon finely chopped fresh
  thyme or ¼ teaspoon dried thyme

¼ teaspoon salt
⅛ teaspoon freshly ground pepper
1 tablespoon olive oil
1 tablespoon finely chopped
  fresh parsley

1. Preheat an oven to 350°F (180°C). Select a baking dish in which the tomatoes will fit in a single layer. Lightly coat with nonstick cooking spray.

2. Arrange the tomatoes in the prepared baking dish. Sprinkle the shallot, garlic, thyme, salt and pepper evenly over the tomatoes and drizzle with the olive oil.

3. Bake until the tomatoes are soft and almost falling apart, 20–22 minutes.

4. To serve, using a slotted spoon, transfer the tomatoes to a serving dish. Sprinkle with the parsley and toss gently to mix.

*Nutritional Analysis
Per Serving:*

**CALORIES 38
(KILOJOULES 160)
PROTEIN 1 G
CARBOHYDRATES 4 G
TOTAL FAT 2 G
SATURATED FAT 0 G
CHOLESTEROL 0 MG
SODIUM 97 MG
DIETARY FIBER 1 G**

Unless they are very watery, you don't have to seed or drain the tomatoes when making this classic accompaniment for broiled or roast poultry or meat. The moisture helps the other ingredients form a savory crust. Use a baking dish that can go from oven to table.

Stuffed Tomatoes

Serves 4

4 large ripe but firm plum (Roma) tomatoes, 1 lb (500 g) total weight, halved lengthwise
¼ teaspoon salt
⅛ teaspoon freshly ground pepper
4 small garlic cloves, peeled and thinly sliced
2 tablespoons olive oil

⅓ cup (¾ oz/20 g) fresh bread crumbs
1 tablespoon finely chopped fresh parsley
1 tablespoon finely chopped fresh basil
1 teaspoon finely chopped fresh thyme leaves or ¼ teaspoon dried thyme

1. Preheat an oven to 400°F (200°C).
2. Arrange the tomatoes, cut sides up, in a 3-qt (3-l) baking dish. Sprinkle with the salt, pepper and garlic. Then drizzle with half of the olive oil.
3. Bake the tomatoes, uncovered, until they are softened and sizzling, 45–60 minutes. Remove from the oven and preheat the broiler (griller).
4. In a small bowl, stir together the bread crumbs, parsley, basil and thyme. Sprinkle the bread crumb mixture over the tomatoes. Drizzle the remaining olive oil over the bread crumb mixture. Broil (grill) until lightly browned, 2–3 minutes.
5. Serve immediately from the baking dish.

Nutritional Analysis Per Serving:

Calories 100
(Kilojoules 421)
Protein 2 g
Carbohydrates 8 g
Total Fat 7 g
Saturated Fat 1 g
Cholesterol 0 mg
Sodium 172 mg
Dietary Fiber 1 g

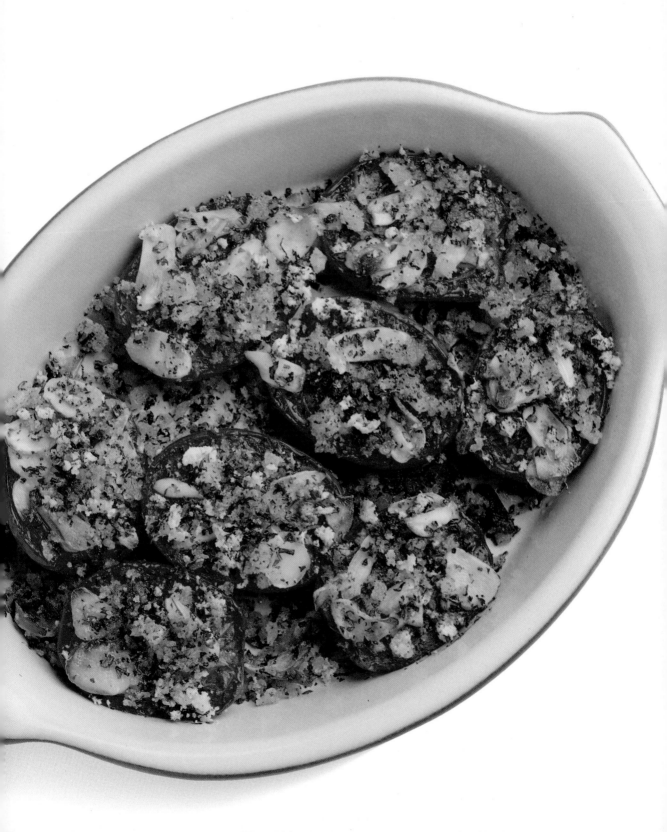

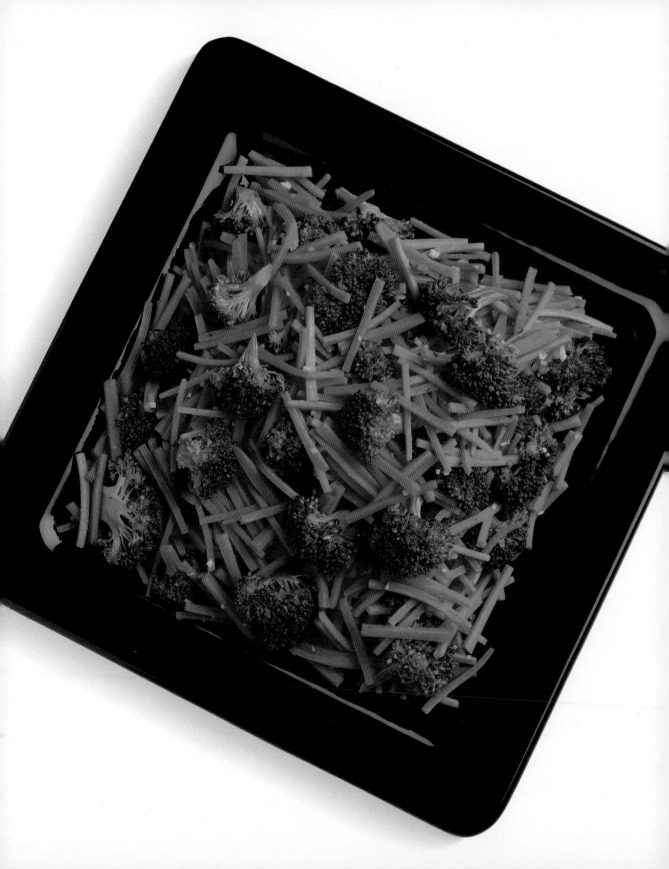

A pair of favorite year-round vegetables come together colorfully in a quick side dish that goes well with anything from steamed fish to roast meat and supplies generous amounts of vitamins A and C. Serve warm or cold.

STIR-FRIED BROCCOLI & CARROTS

Serves 6

2 tablespoons olive oil
4 cups (8 oz/250 g) broccoli florets (from 1 large head)
1 lb (500 g) carrots, peeled and cut into strips
2 garlic cloves, peeled and minced
⅛ teaspoon red pepper flakes, crushed
⅓ cup (3 fl oz/80 ml) Chicken Stock *(recipe on page 127)* or water
½ teaspoon salt

1. In a large, deep frying pan or wok over medium-high heat, warm the olive oil. Add the broccoli and carrots and toss every 15–20 seconds until just beginning to soften, 2–3 minutes. Add the garlic and red pepper flakes and toss for 1 minute longer.
2. Add the Chicken Stock or water and cover. Reduce the heat to medium-low and cook until just tender, 5–6 minutes. Add the salt and toss to mix well.
3. To serve, transfer to a serving dish.

Nutritional Analysis Per Serving:

CALORIES 83
(KILOJOULES 347)
PROTEIN 2 G
CARBOHYDRATES 9 G
TOTAL FAT 5 G
SATURATED FAT 1 G
CHOLESTEROL 0 MG
SODIUM 232 MG
DIETARY FIBER 3 G

Among the most aromatic of herbs, fresh dill provides a unifying
element for this bright medley of vegetables, all of which are rich in vitamin A.
Try this side dish with baked fish or roast lamb.

DILLED CARROTS & SQUASHES

Serves 6

3 carrots, peeled, halved
   lengthwise and sliced
2 tablespoons olive oil
1 small red (Spanish) onion,
   thinly sliced
3 zucchini (courgettes), halved
   lengthwise and sliced
3 yellow summer squash, halved
   lengthwise and sliced
1 garlic clove, peeled and minced
½ teaspoon salt
⅛ teaspoon freshly ground pepper
1 tablespoon chopped fresh dill

1. Fill a saucepan three-fourths full of water, place over medium-high heat and bring to a boil. Add the carrots and boil for 1 minute. Drain in a colander.
2. In a sauté or frying pan over medium heat, warm the olive oil. Add the onion and sauté, stirring occasionally, until slightly softened, 3–5 minutes. Do not allow to brown. Add the carrots and sauté for 1 minute longer. Add the zucchini, yellow squash and garlic and stir to mix well. Cover and cook until all the vegetables are tender-crisp, 2–3 minutes.
3. Add the salt, pepper and dill and stir to mix well.
4. To serve, transfer to a serving bowl.

*Nutritional Analysis
Per Serving:*

CALORIES 103
(KILOJOULES 431)
PROTEIN 3 G
CARBOHYDRATES 14 G
TOTAL FAT 5 G
SATURATED FAT 1 G
CHOLESTEROL 0 MG
SODIUM 203 MG
DIETARY FIBER 3 G

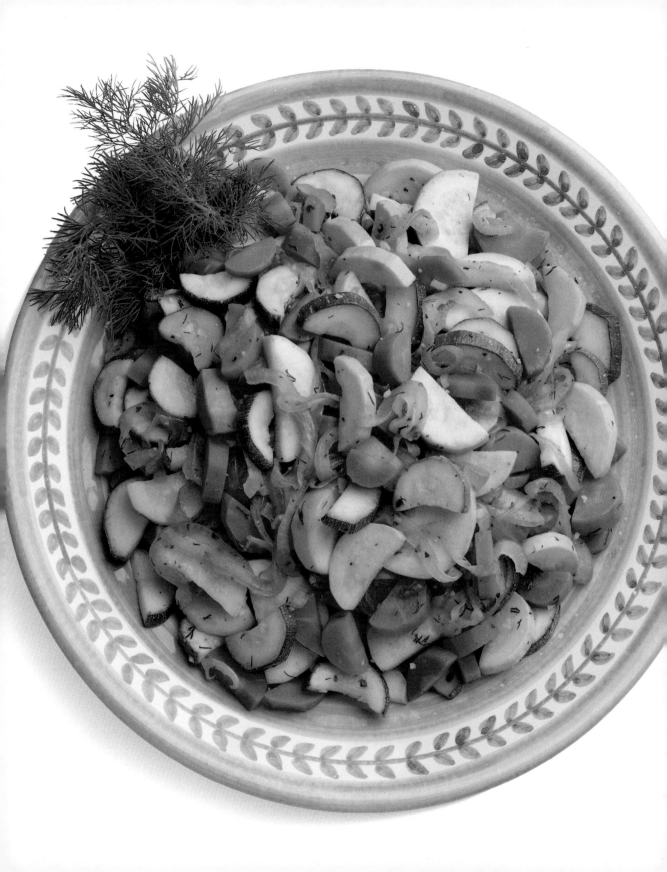

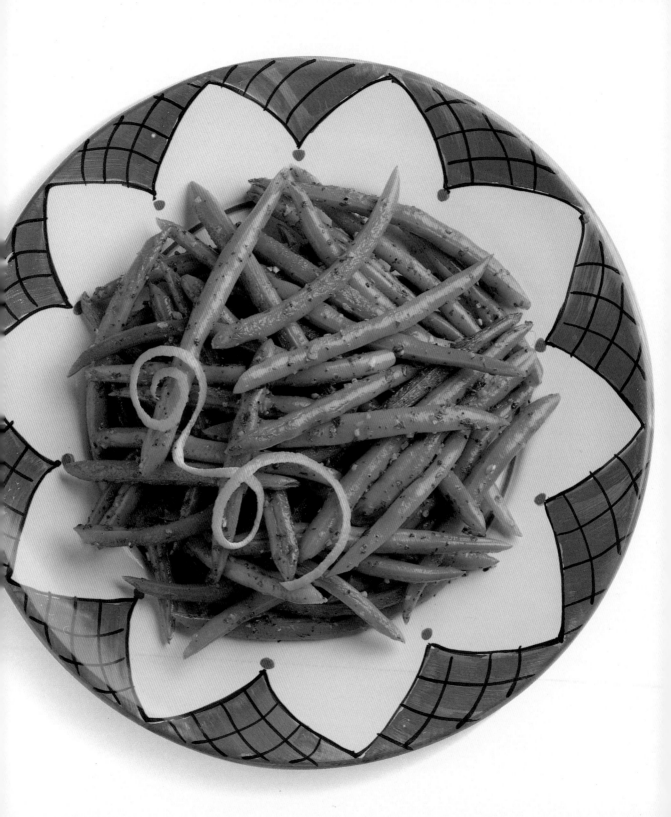

Rich in the classic flavors of French cooking, this side dish is exceptionally easy.
In fact, you can boil the green beans up to 6 hours in advance, refrigerate them wrapped
in paper towels and simply return to room temperature before continuing.

LEMONY GREEN BEANS

Serves 4

1 lb (500 g) small green beans
1½ tablespoons olive oil
1 garlic clove, peeled and minced
1 shallot, peeled and
  finely chopped

2 tablespoons finely chopped
  fresh parsley
1 teaspoon fresh lemon juice
¼ teaspoon salt
⅛ teaspoon freshly ground pepper

1. Fill a saucepan three-fourths full of water, place over medium-high heat and bring to a boil. Add the beans and cook until tender but still slightly resistant when pierced with a fork, 5–6 minutes. Drain the beans in a colander and rinse with cool water to stop the cooking and preserve the color. Drain again.
2. In a sauté or frying pan over medium heat, warm the olive oil. Add the beans, stir well to coat with the oil and raise the heat to high. Sauté, stirring occasionally, until lightly browned, 2–3 minutes. Add the garlic, shallot, parsley and lemon juice and sauté 30 seconds longer. Remove from the heat, add the salt and pepper and stir to mix well.
3. To serve, transfer to a serving dish.

Nutritional Analysis Per Serving:

**CALORIES 80
(KILOJOULES 334)
PROTEIN 2 G
CARBOHYDRATES 8 G
TOTAL FAT 5 G
SATURATED FAT 1 G
CHOLESTEROL 0 MG
SODIUM 142 MG
DIETARY FIBER 2 G**

Just a little orange and lemon juice, added to the braising liquid, complement the deep flavor of beets, while slightly balancing their inherent sweetness. This side dish goes especially well with roast chicken or beef.

Rosy Beets in Citrus Glaze

Serves 4

6 beets, peeled and cut into wedges
¾ cup (6 fl oz/180 ml) Chicken Stock *(recipe on page 127)* or water
2 tablespoons fresh lemon juice
3 tablespoons fresh orange juice
1 tablespoon olive oil
1 tablespoon finely chopped fresh parsley
⅛ teaspoon freshly ground pepper

1. In a heavy, nonreactive saucepan over medium heat, combine the beets, Chicken Stock or water, lemon and orange juices and olive oil. Bring to a simmer, reduce the heat to low, cover partially and braise, tossing every 10 minutes, until tender when pierced with a fork and glazed with the liquid, 40–45 minutes.
2. Add the parsley and pepper and toss to coat well.
3. To serve, transfer to a serving bowl.

Nutritional Analysis Per Serving:

Calories 97
(Kilojoules 407)
Protein 2 g
Carbohydrates 15 g
Total Fat 4 g
Saturated Fat 1 g
Cholesterol 0 mg
Sodium 149 mg
Dietary Fiber 1 g

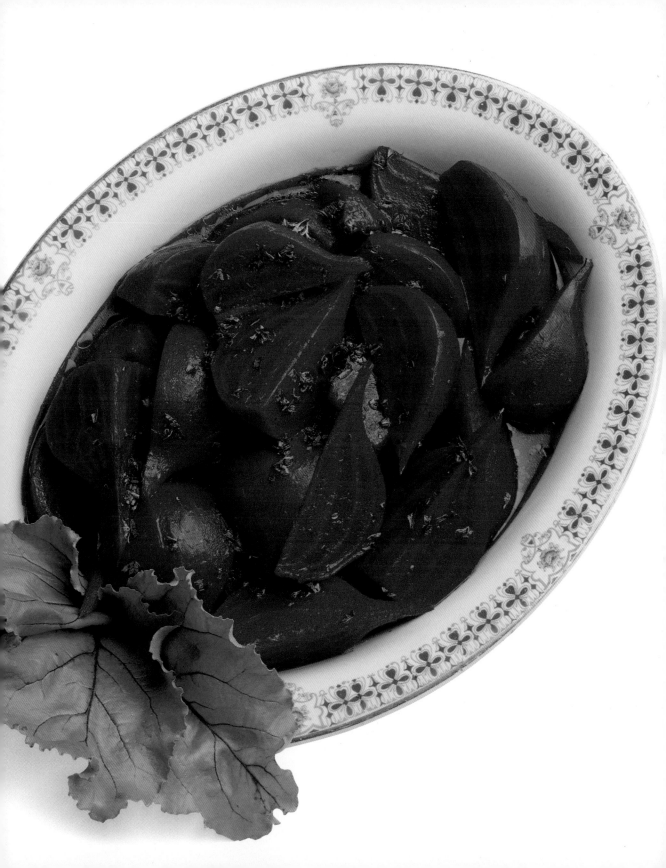

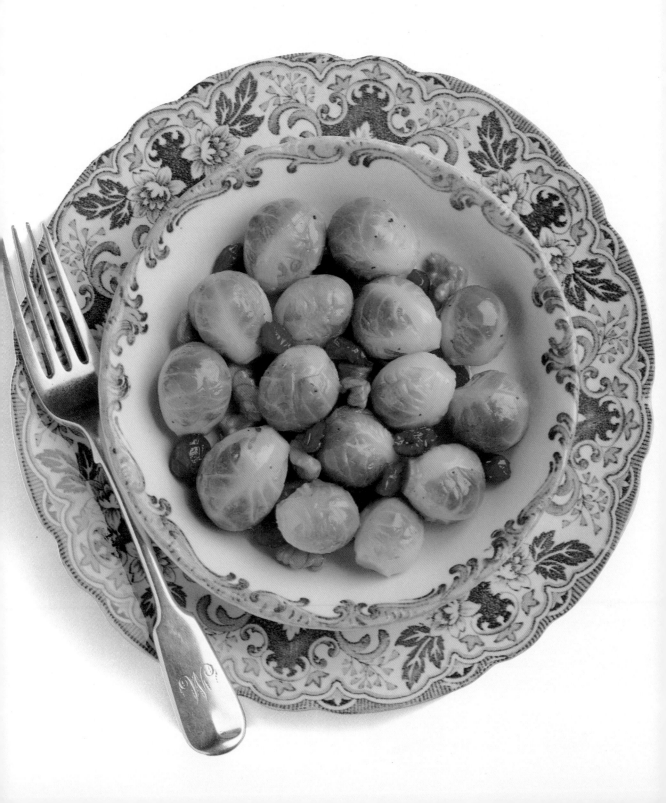

Brussels sprouts taste wonderfully fresh and crisp when just briefly steamed. Seek out the smallest, most tender sprouts for this recipe. Frozen vegetables can be used when sprouts are out of season. If pomegranates are unavailable, substitute dried cranberries.

Steamed Brussels Sprouts & Walnuts

Serves 6

1½ lb (750 g) Brussels sprouts
1 tablespoon red wine vinegar
1 teaspoon balsamic vinegar
⅛ teaspoon salt
⅛ teaspoon freshly ground pepper
2 tablespoons walnut oil

1 tablespoon boiling water
2 tablespoons shelled walnuts,
  toasted and coarsely chopped
½ cup (2 oz/60 g) fresh pomegranate
  seeds (from 1 pomegranate) or
  dried cranberries, optional

1. Trim the stem ends of each Brussels sprout slightly to release the bitter outer leaves. Discard the leaves. Cut a shallow cross in the stem end of each sprout.
2. Pour water to a depth of 1 inch (2.5 cm) in a steamer pan. Put the steamer rack in place and the sprouts on the rack. Cover and bring to a boil. Steam over medium heat until tender when pierced with a fork, 8–10 minutes. Place under cool running water to stop the cooking and preserve the color. Drain well.
3. To make the vinaigrette, in a small bowl, whisk together the red wine and balsamic vinegars, salt and pepper. Add the walnut oil in a thin, steady stream, whisking continuously, until well blended. Whisk in the boiling water.
4. Place the Brussels sprouts in a serving bowl. Drizzle with the vinaigrette and toss to coat well. Add the walnuts, toss again, and let stand at room temperature for at least 2 hours or for up to 4 hours. Stir occasionally to make sure all the sprouts are equally coated with the vinaigrette.
5. To serve, sprinkle with the pomegranate seeds or cranberries, if using.

Nutritional Analysis Per Serving:

Calories 101
(Kilojoules 424)
Protein 4 g
Carbohydrates 10 g
Total Fat 6 g
Saturated Fat 1 g
Cholesterol 0 mg
Sodium 72 mg
Dietary Fiber 6 g

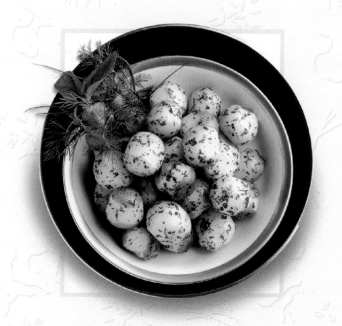

Potatoes

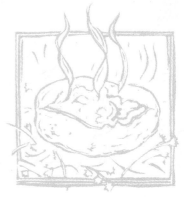

$\mathcal{N}$ative to South America, the potato has been a food source since prehistoric times. Now cultivated worldwide, this humble-seeming vegetable is the workhorse of a well-balanced diet. While at one time not considered a healthy food, it is what was combined with the potatoes—not the potatoes themselves—that produced high calorie and fat numbers. Potatoes actually have high fiber content and provide good-quality complex carbohydrates. And their taste, texture and the vast number of varieties available make potatoes adaptable to many cooking methods and seasoning styles. With that in mind, this chapter offers cooking techniques, including potatoes baked until crusty with Gruyère cheese or mashed to an appealing richness with lowfat buttermilk, plus seasoning and garnishing ideas— especially with herbs—that show methods for achieving flavor and texture without adding fat or sodium. Using these ingredients and techniques allow you to put generous helpings of potato on the table whenever desired.

New potatoes, whether the red or white varieties, have a distinctive tenderness that is nicely accentuated by steaming. To complement their flavor, select a green-hued extra-virgin olive oil with a fruity taste.

HERBED NEW POTATOES

Serves 4

1½ lb (750 g) small new potatoes, well scrubbed and unpeeled

2 tablespoons extra-virgin olive oil

1 tablespoon finely chopped fresh dill

2 teaspoons finely chopped fresh chives

2 teaspoons finely chopped fresh basil

¼ teaspoon salt

⅛ teaspoon white pepper

1. Using a sharp knife, peel a ring of skin from around the center of each potato.

2. Pour water to a depth of 1 inch (2.5 cm) in a steamer pan. Put the steamer rack in place and put the potatoes on the rack. Cover and bring the water to a boil. Steam over medium heat until tender when pierced with a fork, 15–20 minutes.

3. Just before the potatoes are done, in a serving bowl, stir together the olive oil, dill, chives, basil, salt and pepper.

4. To serve, transfer the cooked potatoes to the serving bowl and toss gently to coat.

Nutritional Analysis Per Serving:

CALORIES 199
(KILOJOULES 835)
PROTEIN 3 G
CARBOHYDRATES 31 G
TOTAL FAT 7 G
SATURATED FAT 1 G
CHOLESTEROL 0 MG
SODIUM 149 MG
DIETARY FIBER 3 G

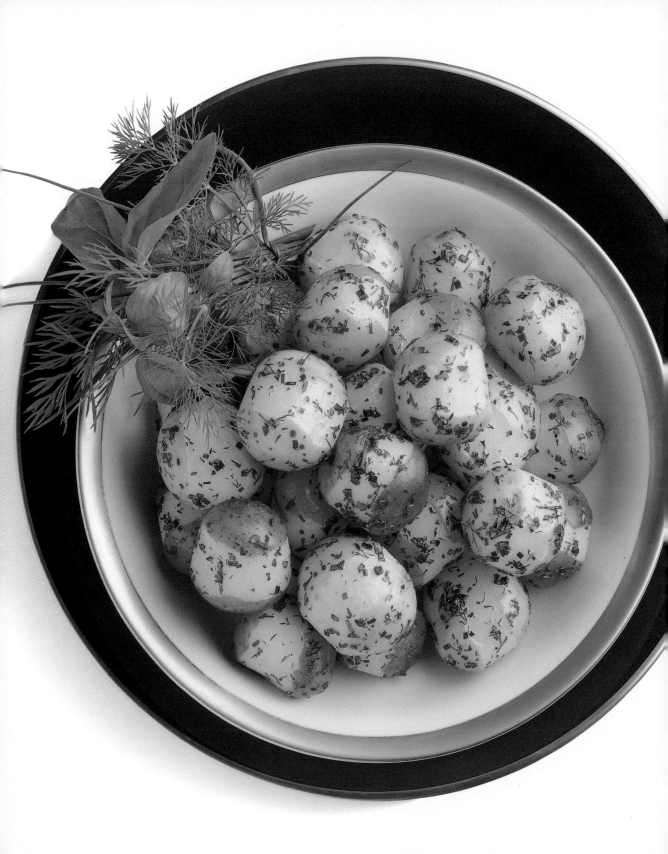

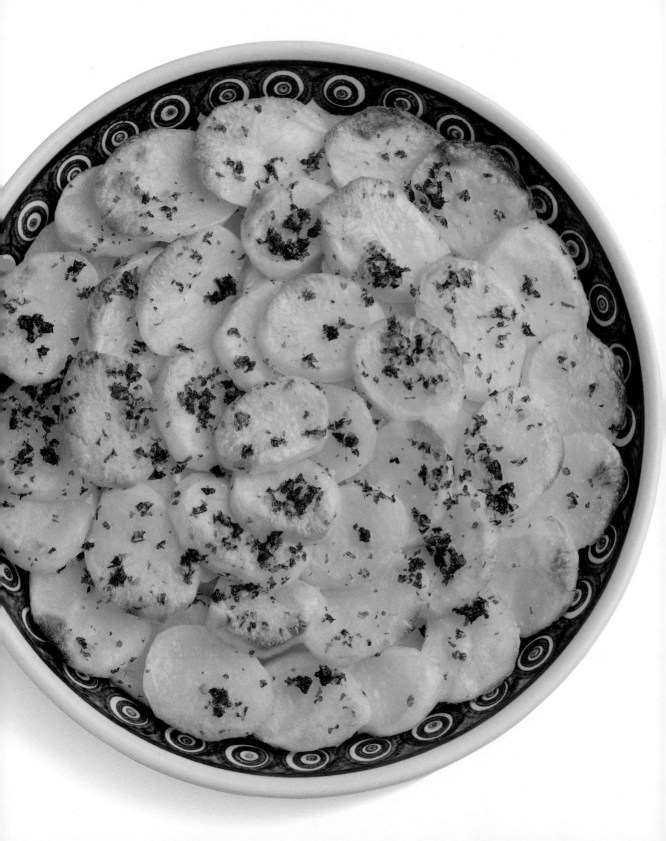

Select an attractive baking dish that will go directly from the oven to the table for this fast version of a classic French dish. Topping the assembled dish with another baking dish of the same size compresses the potatoes into a cakelike consistency.

QUICK POTATOES ANNA

Serves 4

2 lb (1 kg) small, waxy, white-fleshed potatoes, peeled and cut crosswise into ¼ inch (6 mm) thick slices
2 tablespoons olive oil

2 garlic cloves, peeled and minced
1 teaspoon salt
¼ teaspoon finely ground white pepper
1 tablespoon finely chopped fresh parsley

1. Preheat an oven to 400°F (200°C). Lightly coat a 9-inch (23-cm) round baking dish with nonstick cooking spray.
2. In a bowl, combine the potato slices, olive oil, garlic, salt and pepper. Toss to coat well.
3. Using a slotted spoon to remove them from the bowl, arrange the potato slices in rows in a circular pattern in the prepared baking dish, starting at the outer edge and overlapping the slices a little. Pour any of the oil mixture remaining in the bowl over the potatoes.
4. Lightly coat a piece of aluminum foil with nonstick cooking spray and lay it, sprayed side down, over the potatoes. Place another baking dish of the same size on the foil, bottom side down, and press down firmly.
5. Bake for 40 minutes and remove the top dish and foil. Continue to bake until the potatoes are tender, browned and crispy, 15–20 minutes longer. Remove the top dish and foil.
6. To serve, sprinkle the parsley over the top.

Nutritional Analysis Per Serving:

CALORIES 229
(KILOJOULES 964)
PROTEIN 4 G
CARBOHYDRATES 37 G
TOTAL FAT 7 G
SATURATED FAT 1 G
CHOLESTEROL 0 MG
SODIUM 567 MG
DIETARY FIBER 3 G

Sautéed leeks and jalapeños are layered with the potatoes in this crusty gratin. Look for the Yukon Gold variety of potatoes for this dish, although any waxy potato will work well. Serve with grilled poultry or meat.

SPICY POTATOES BOULANGÈRE

Serves 6

1 tablespoon plus 3 teaspoons olive oil

1 leek, green and white parts, finely chopped

3 garlic cloves, peeled and minced

2 tablespoons finely chopped fresh parsley

1½ cups (6 oz/185 g) grated Gruyère cheese

½ teaspoon salt

¼ teaspoon freshly ground pepper

2½ lb (1.25 kg) waxy, yellow- or white-fleshed potatoes, well scrubbed, unpeeled and sliced crosswise

1 fresh jalapeño pepper, seeded and minced

1 cup (8 fl oz/250 ml) Chicken Stock *(recipe on page 127)* or water

1. In a sauté or frying pan over medium heat, warm the 1 tablespoon of olive oil. Add the leek and sauté, stirring, until softened, 4–5 minutes. Remove from the heat.

2. Preheat an oven to 375°F (190°C). Coat a 3-qt (3-l) baking dish with nonstick cooking spray.

3. In a small bowl, combine the garlic, parsley, Gruyère cheese, salt, pepper and leeks.

4. Arrange one-third of the potato slices in the bottom of the prepared dish. Sprinkle with one-third of the leek mixture, and then one-half of the minced jalapeño. Drizzle with 1 teaspoon of the olive oil. Layer half of the remaining potatoes on top, sprinkle with half of the remaining leek mixture and all of the remaining jalapeño. Layer the remaining potatoes on top. Pour the Chicken Stock or water evenly over the potatoes and sprinkle with the remaining leek mixture. Drizzle the remaining 2 teaspoons of olive oil over the top.

5. Coat one side of a sheet of aluminum foil large enough to cover the baking dish with nonstick cooking spray. Place over

Nutritional Analysis Per Serving:

CALORIES 330

(KILOJOULES 1,387)

PROTEIN 13 G

CARBOHYDRATES 38 G

TOTAL FAT 14 G

SATURATED FAT 6 G

CHOLESTEROL 31 MG

SODIUM 350 MG

DIETARY FIBER 4 G

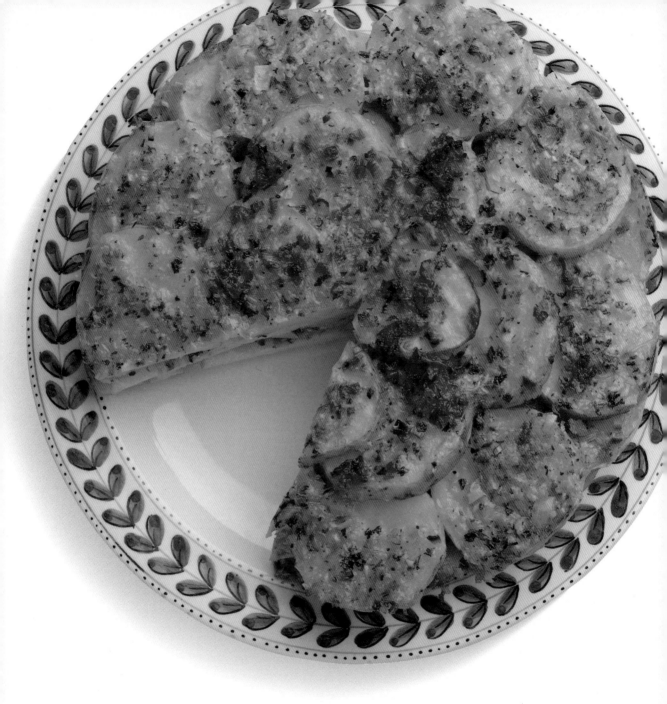

the dish, sprayed side down, crimping the edges to secure
in place. Bake for 30 minutes. Remove the foil and continue
baking until the top is brown and crusty and the potatoes are
tender when pierced with a fork, 30–40 minutes longer.

6. To serve, cool for 5 minutes before transferring to a serving
platter, cutting into wedges and placing onto individual plates.

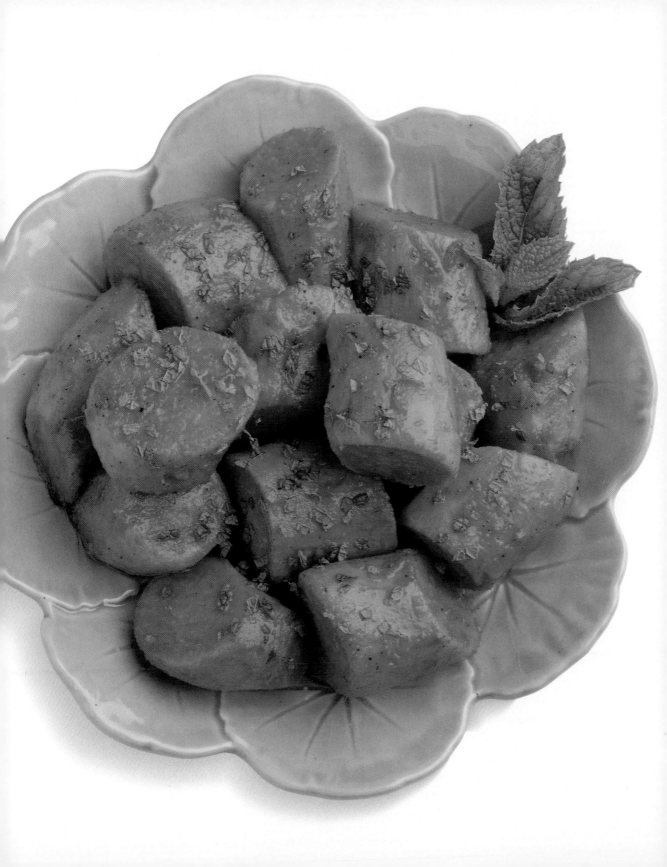

The syrupy glaze that cloaks these sweet potatoes turns them into an ideal accompaniment to roast poultry and a fitting addition to a holiday table. This preparation is a great way to get children to eat their vegetables.

ORANGE-GLAZED SWEET POTATOES

Serves 6

3 sweet potatoes, ½ lb (250 g) each, well scrubbed, unpeeled and pierced with a fork
⅓ cup (3 fl oz/80 ml) orange juice
1 teaspoon finely grated orange zest
3 tablespoons firmly packed dark brown sugar

1 tablespoon olive oil
½ teaspoon ground ginger
¼ teaspoon ground allspice
⅛ teaspoon ground nutmeg
½ teaspoon finely chopped fresh mint

1. Preheat an oven to 400°F (200°C).
2. Place each sweet potato on a square of aluminum foil large enough to enclose it completely. Wrap the foil around the sweet potatoes and seal the edges securely. Bake until tender, about 45 minutes. Remove from the oven, unwrap and let cool slightly. When cool enough to handle, peel the sweet potatoes and cut into 2-inch (5-cm) chunks.
3. While the sweet potatoes are baking, in a large saucepan over medium-high heat, combine the orange juice, orange zest, brown sugar, olive oil, ginger, allspice and nutmeg. Cook continuously, swirling the pan, until the mixture reduces to a syrupy glaze, 3–4 minutes. Remove from the heat and set aside until the sweet potatoes are ready.
4. Add the sweet potato chunks to the pan holding the glaze, cover and place over very low heat. Cook, shaking the pan occasionally to keep the potatoes from scorching, until the potatoes are tender when pierced with a fork, 3–4 minutes.
5. To serve, transfer to a serving bowl and sprinkle with the mint.

Nutritional Analysis Per Serving:

CALORIES 139
(KILOJOULES 584)
PROTEIN 1 G
CARBOHYDRATES 28 G
TOTAL FAT 3 G
SATURATED FAT 0 G
CHOLESTEROL 0 MG
SODIUM 14 MG
DIETARY FIBER 2 G

Stuffed potatoes combine in one tidy package all the pleasures of both mashed and baked potatoes. This side dish can be prepared hours ahead and baked just before serving, making it an ideal choice for entertaining.

LEEK & PARMESAN STUFFED POTATOES

Serves 8

4 baking potatoes, about ½ lb (250 g) each, well scrubbed, unpeeled and pierced with a fork

4 teaspoons plus 1 tablespoon olive oil

1 leek, green and white parts, finely chopped

⅔ cup (5 fl oz/160 ml) lowfat milk, warmed

¼ cup (1 oz/30 g) plus 2 teaspoons freshly grated Parmesan cheese

½ teaspoon salt

⅛ teaspoon white pepper

2 teaspoons finely chopped fresh parsley

Nutritional Analysis Per Serving:

CALORIES 167

(KILOJOULES 701)

PROTEIN 5 G

CARBOHYDRATES 22 G

TOTAL FAT 6 G

SATURATED FAT 2 G

CHOLESTEROL 7 MG

SODIUM 279 MG

DIETARY FIBER 2 G

1. Preheat an oven to 425°F (220°C). Rub each potato all over with 1 teaspoon of the olive oil.

2. Place the potatoes on an ungreased baking sheet and bake until tender, about 1 hour. Set aside until cool enough to handle. Reduce the oven to 400°F (200°C).

3. While the potatoes are cooking, in a small frying pan over medium heat, warm the remaining 1 tablespoon olive oil. Add the leek and sauté, stirring occasionally, until softened but not browned, 4–5 minutes.

4. Using a sharp knife, cut each cooked potato in half lengthwise and scoop out the potato pulp from each half, leaving only a thin shell. Place the pulp in a bowl and mash it with a potato masher or fork.

5. Add the warm milk, the ¼ cup (1 oz/30 g) Parmesan cheese, sautéed leek, salt and pepper to the mashed potatoes. Stir vigorously to mix well.

6. Dividing the potato mixture evenly, spoon it back into the potato shells, mounding the tops attractively. Sprinkle an even amount of the remaining 2 teaspoons Parmesan cheese over the top of each potato half. Place the stuffed potatoes in an attractive baking dish that can go directly to the table. Bake until the potatoes are hot and the cheese is melted and bubbling, 10–15 minutes.

7. To serve, sprinkle with the parsley.

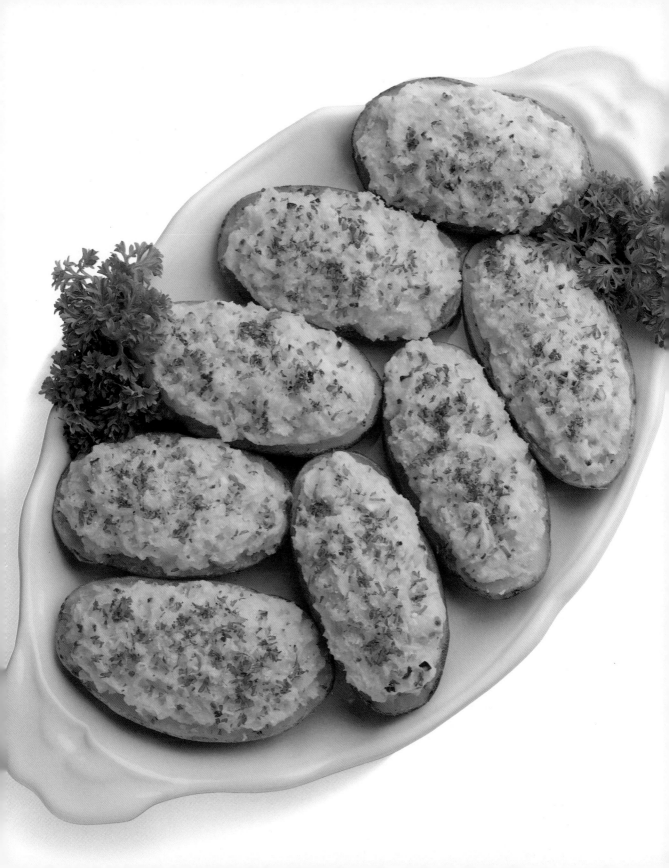

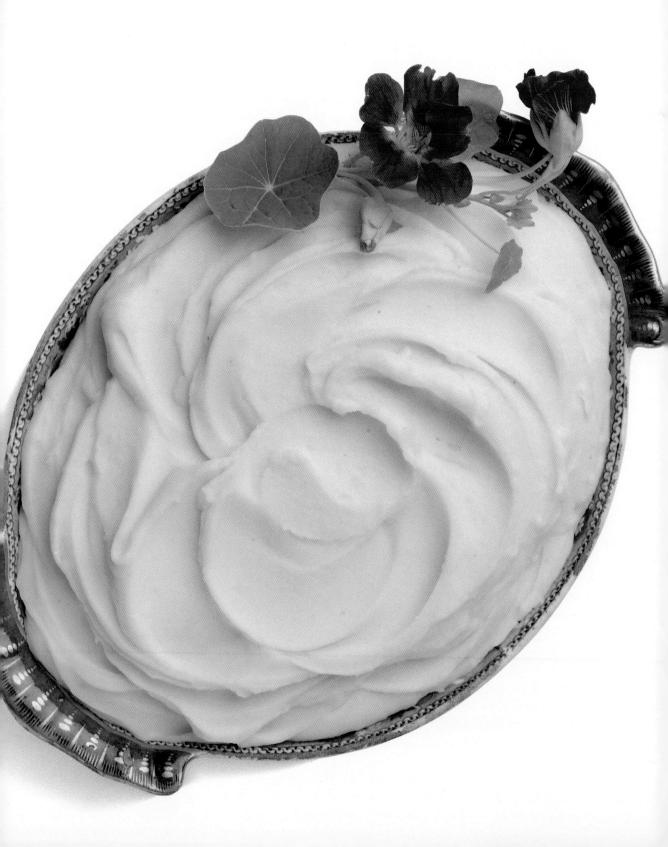

This old-fashioned favorite becomes as healthy as it is comforting by using lowfat buttermilk in place of milk and butter. Use brown-skinned baking potatoes for fluffy results. Garnish with edible nasturtium flowers, if desired.

Buttermilk Mashed Potatoes

Serves 6

2 lb (1 kg) baking potatoes, peeled and cut into chunks
¼ teaspoon salt
1 tablespoon olive oil

¾ cup (6 fl oz/180 ml) lowfat buttermilk, warmed
white pepper

1. To remove excess starch, immerse the potatoes in cold water to cover for 5 minutes and drain in a colander. Fill a large saucepan three-fourths full of water and bring to a boil. Add the salt and potatoes and cook until tender when pierced with a fork, 15–20 minutes.

2. Drain the potatoes in a colander. Return them to the pan and cook over high heat to dry, turning constantly to prevent scorching, until all the moisture evaporates, 1–2 minutes.

3. Using a potato masher or fork, mash the potatoes. Add the olive oil and slowly add the warm buttermilk, stirring constantly with a large spoon until thoroughly combined. Add the white pepper to taste and stir to mix well.

4. To serve, transfer to a serving bowl.

Nutritional Analysis Per Serving:

**Calories 122
(Kilojoules 512)
Protein 3 g
Carbohydrates 22 g
Total Fat 3 g
Saturated Fat 0 g
Cholesterol 1 mg
Sodium 129 mg
Dietary Fiber 2 g**

Baking in parchment paper—what the French call *en papillote*—produces tender, flavorful results with minimal fat. For more flavor, drizzle 1 teaspoon of dry white wine over the contents of each packet before sealing.

POTATOES IN PARCHMENT

Serves 6

18 very small new potatoes,
    1½ oz (45 g) each, well
    scrubbed and unpeeled
4½ teaspoons olive oil
½ teaspoon salt
¼ teaspoon freshly ground pepper
2 tablespoons finely chopped
    fresh dill
3 thin lemon slices, halved
6 fresh dill sprigs

1. Preheat an oven to 450°F (230°C). Cut out 6 pieces of parchment paper, each 6 inches (15 cm) square. Fold each square in half, and then open out flat again.

2. Place 3 potatoes on one half of each square. Sprinkle an equal amount of the olive oil, salt, pepper and dill over the potatoes in each packet. Top each with a halved lemon slice.

3. Fold the uncovered side of the parchment over the potatoes to cover completely and crimp the edges to make an airtight seal. Fold over the ends to securely close each packet. Carefully transfer the packets to a baking sheet.

4. Bake until the packets are puffed and golden, 30–35 minutes.

5. To serve, place each packet on an individual plate, tear open and slip in a dill sprig.

Nutritional Analysis Per Serving:

CALORIES 102
(KILOJOULES 427)
PROTEIN 2 G
CARBOHYDRATES 16 G
TOTAL FAT 4 G
SATURATED FAT 0 G
CHOLESTEROL 0 MG
SODIUM 190 MG
DIETARY FIBER 1 G

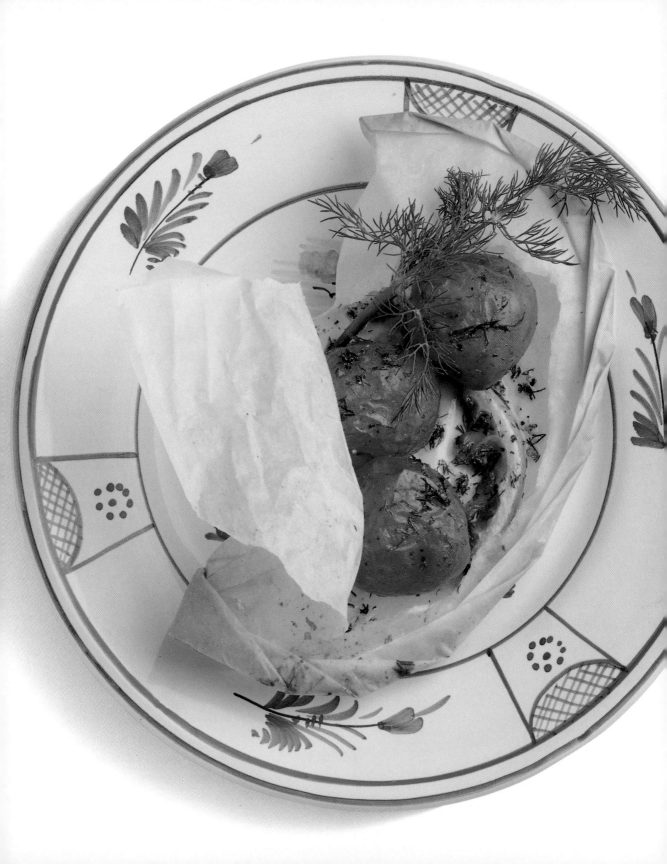

With the widespread availability of zucchini and peppers, you can bake this Mediterranean-inspired side dish anytime. Use as part of a dinner party, buffet entry or serve as a vegetarian main dish for four.

Ratatouille-Potato Gratin

Serves 8

2 tablespoons olive oil
1 leek, green and white parts, finely chopped
1 red bell pepper (capsicum), seeded, deribbed and cut into strips
2 zucchini (courgettes), thinly sliced
1 lb (500 g) ripe but firm tomatoes, peeled, seeded and coarsely chopped
2 garlic cloves, peeled and minced
½ teaspoon salt
¼ teaspoon freshly ground pepper

1 teaspoon finely chopped fresh thyme or ½ teaspoon dried thyme
4 tablespoons finely chopped fresh basil
2 lb (1 kg) baking potatoes, peeled and cut into ¼ inch (6 mm) thick slices
½ cup (2 oz/60 g) freshly grated Parmesan cheese

1. Preheat an oven to 400°F (200°C). Coat a deep 3-qt (3-l) baking dish that can go directly to the table with nonstick cooking spray.

2. In a large sauté or frying pan over medium heat, warm the olive oil. Add the leek and sauté, stirring occasionally, until soft but not brown, 4–5 minutes. Add the bell pepper and zucchini and sauté, stirring occasionally, until slightly softened, about 3 minutes longer.

3. Add the tomatoes and raise the heat to medium-high. Sauté, stirring, until the excess moisture from the tomatoes evaporates, 3–5 minutes. Add the garlic, salt, pepper, thyme and half of the basil and stir to mix well. Remove from the heat.

4. Arrange half of the potatoes in the prepared dish, overlapping the slices. Spread half of the sautéed vegetable mixture over the potatoes and then sprinkle evenly with half of the Parmesan cheese. Repeat with the remaining potatoes, vegetable mixture and cheese. Cover tightly with aluminum foil.

Nutritional Analysis Per Serving:

Calories 171
(Kilojoules 720)
Protein 6 g
Carbohydrates 22 g
Total Fat 7 g
Saturated Fat 2 g
Cholesterol 5 mg
Sodium 265 mg
Dietary Fiber 3 g

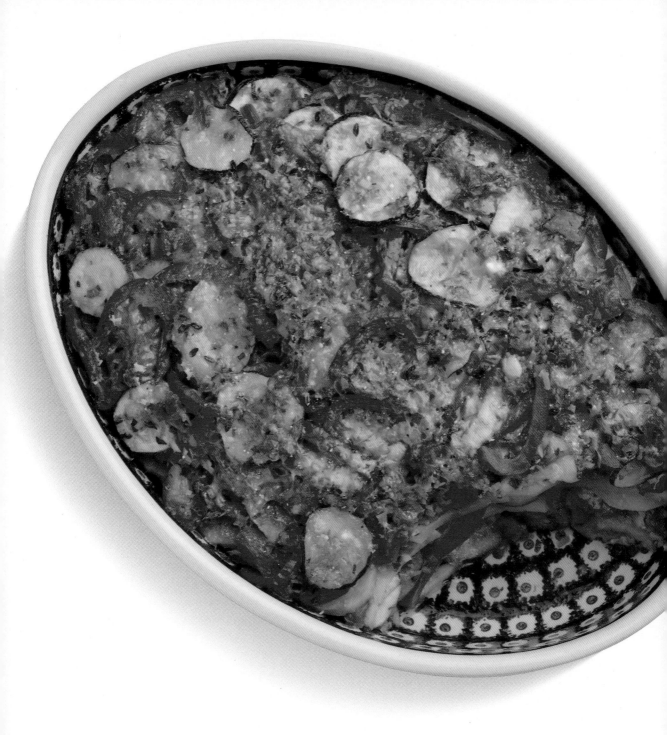

5. Bake for 45 minutes. Remove the foil and bake until
the potatoes are tender and the top is nicely browned,
30–40 minutes longer.

6. To serve, sprinkle with the remaining basil.

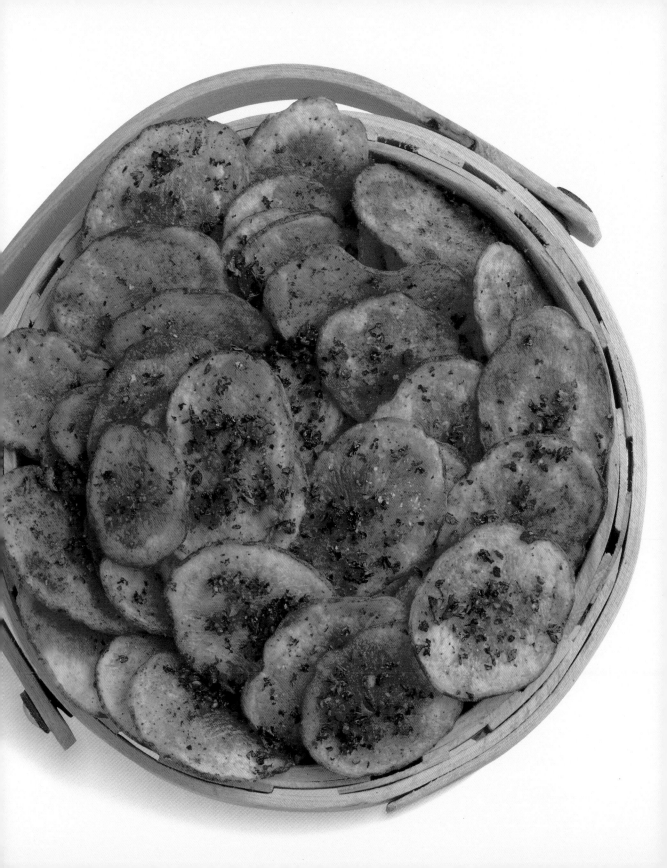

Spraying thin slices of potato with nonstick cooking spray and baking them produces crisp chips with virtually none of the fat possessed by deep-fried versions. Experiment with different types of potatoes and various herb combinations for different flavors.

SPICY POTATO CHIPS

Serves 6

2 lb (1 kg) baking potatoes, well
   scrubbed, unpeeled and cut
   into ⅛ inch (3 mm) thick slices
½ teaspoon salt
¼ teaspoon freshly ground pepper
½ garlic clove, peeled and
   finely minced

¼ teaspoon paprika
⅛ teaspoon cayenne pepper
¼ teaspoon coarsely cracked
   black pepper
1 teaspoon chopped fresh parsley

1. Preheat an oven to 400°F (200°C). Lightly coat 2 nonstick baking sheets with nonstick cooking spray.
2. Place the potatoes in a shallow bowl and coat lightly with nonstick cooking spray. Sprinkle with the salt and ground pepper.
3. Arrange the potato slices in a single layer on the prepared baking sheets. Bake until crispy brown, 20–25 minutes.
4. While the potatoes are cooking, in a large bowl, stir together the garlic, paprika, cayenne pepper, cracked pepper and parsley.
5. When the potatoes are done, add them to the bowl and toss gently to coat.
6. To serve, transfer to a basket.

*Nutritional Analysis
Per Serving:*

CALORIES 118
(KILOJOULES 494)
PROTEIN 3 G
CARBOHYDRATES 25 G
TOTAL FAT 1 G
SATURATED FAT 0 G
CHOLESTEROL 0 MG
SODIUM 375 MG
DIETARY FIBER 3 G

A clever but easy cutting technique gives these oven-baked potatoes their unusual shape and name. Blanching the potatoes before they go into the oven helps ensure even cooking. The small amount of oil keeps fat low while the herbs keep flavor high.

ROASTED ACCORDION POTATOES

Serves 6

6 large red or white potatoes,
   about ½ lb (250 g) each
2 tablespoons olive oil
½ teaspoon salt
⅛ teaspoon freshly ground pepper
2 tablespoons freshly grated
   Romano cheese
2 teaspoons finely chopped
   fresh chives
2 teaspoons finely chopped
   fresh parsley

*Nutritional Analysis
Per Serving:*

CALORIES 214
(KILOJOULES 899)
PROTEIN 4 G
CARBOHYDRATES 37 G
TOTAL FAT 6 G
SATURATED FAT 1 G
CHOLESTEROL 2 MG
SODIUM 218 MG
DIETARY FIBER 3 G

1. Preheat an oven to 425°F (220°C).

2. Peel the potatoes and immerse them in a bowl of cold water to cover to prevent them from darkening.

3. Fill a saucepan three-fourths full of water and bring to a boil. Drain the potatoes, add them to the pan. Boil for 5 minutes. Drain well and dry thoroughly with a kitchen towel.

4. Run a skewer through each potato so that it rests about one fourth from the bottom of the potato and three fourths from the top. Using a sharp knife and starting ½ inch (12 mm) from the end of a potato, cut down through the upper part of the potato at ⅛-inch (3-mm) intervals just until you hit the skewer. The potatoes will then resemble a fan or an accordion when cooked.

5. Coat a baking dish just large enough to hold all the potatoes side by side with nonstick cooking spray. Arrange the potatoes, fan side up, in the dish and brush evenly with the olive oil. Be sure that all the exposed surfaces are coated. If the potatoes will not stand upright, trim off a slice from the bottom to make a flat base. Sprinkle with the salt and pepper.

6. Bake until barely tender when pierced with a fork, 30–45 minutes. The timing will depend upon the size of the potatoes. Sprinkle the Romano cheese evenly over the potatoes and continue to bake until crispy and golden, 10–15 minutes longer.

7. To serve, transfer to a serving platter and garnish with the chives and parsley.

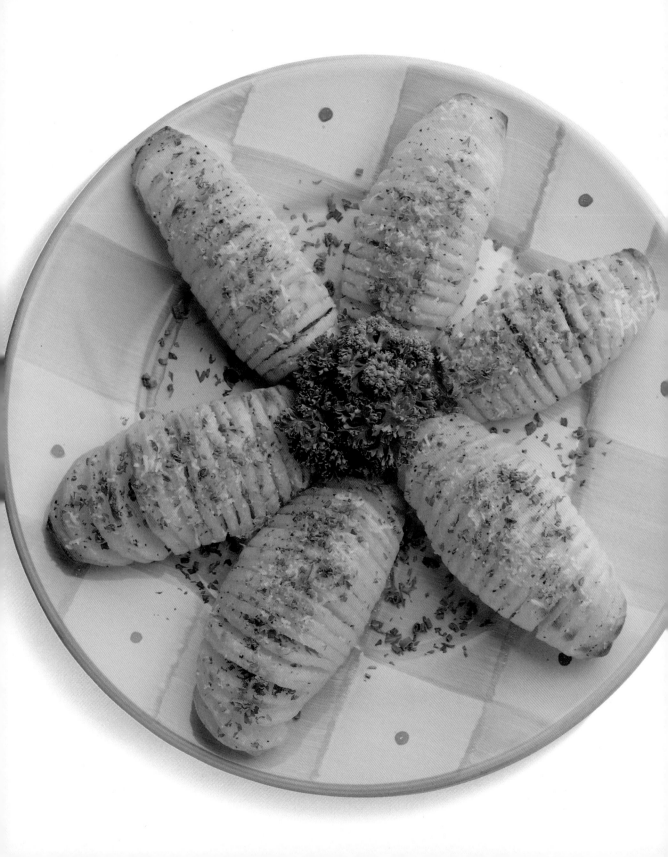

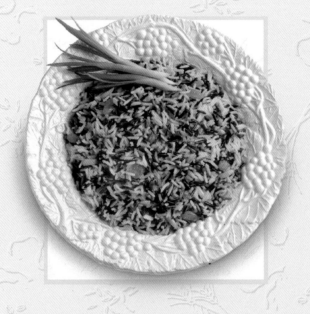

Rice, Beans & Grains

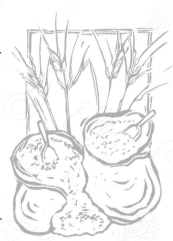

With more than 7,000 types of rice grown worldwide, it is no wonder that it is the main food source for half the planet's population. The other half of the people of the world use a combination of potatoes or beans and grains as their diet staple. This chapter only begins to tap the wondrous variety of these high-fiber products. Recipes including saffron-flavored rice, black beans topped with spicy salsa, and polenta with herbed pesto are eye-opening for their wide array of seasonings and embellishments. These good food combinations and the healthy cooking techniques described on the following pages show that everyday foods can be enlivened to great effect without the addition of excessive calories, fat or sodium. Dispelling the notion that rice, bean and grain dishes need be mild foils for extravagant main dishes, these recipes prove that by using seasonal produce and mastering simple cooking techniques, side dishes become equal partners in a well-balanced meal. In fact, these flavorful side dishes can easily move to center stage for lunch and other light meals.

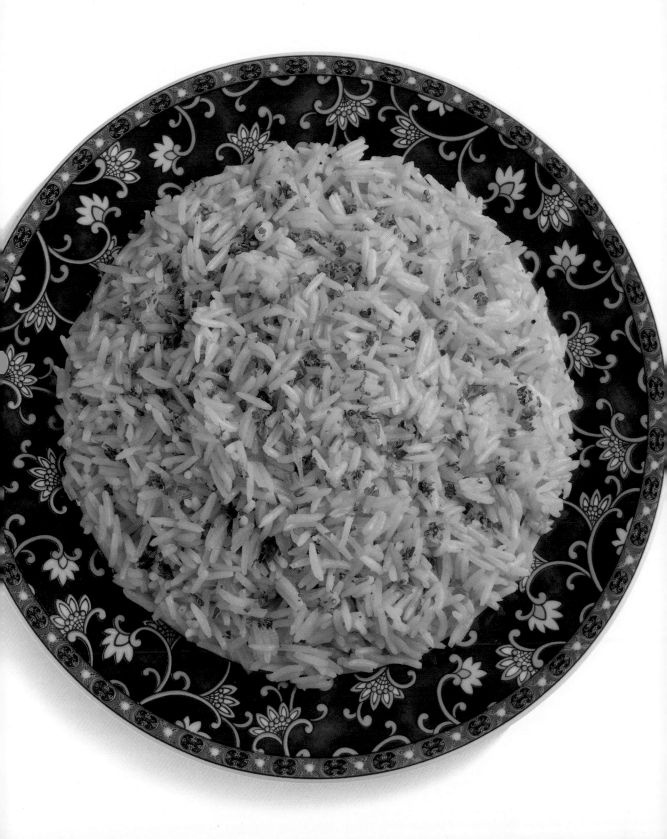

The resulting golden rice, brightly flecked with green, makes an excellent accompaniment to poached sole or orange roughy. The dried stigmas of a crocus, saffron is one of the most expensive spices in the world; however, a little of it goes a long way.

SAFFRON RICE

Serves 6

¼ teaspoon saffron threads or
⅛ teaspoon powdered saffron
2 cups (16 fl oz/500 ml) Chicken
Stock *(recipe on page 127)* or water
2 tablespoons olive oil
2 green (spring) onions, green and
white parts, finely chopped

1 cup (7 oz/220 g) long-grain
white rice
½ teaspoon salt
¼ teaspoon freshly ground pepper
1 tablespoon finely chopped
fresh parsley

1. If using saffron threads, in a saucepan over medium heat, warm the Chicken Stock or water. When it is hot to the touch, add the saffron threads, remove from the heat and let stand for 20 minutes. If using powdered saffron, skip this step and add it with the salt and pepper in step 3.

2. In a sauté or deep frying pan over medium-low heat, warm the olive oil. Add the green onions and sauté, stirring, until softened but not browned, 1–2 minutes. Add the rice and stir to coat thoroughly with the oil. Continue cooking over medium-low heat, stirring occasionally, until the rice just begins to brown lightly, 3–4 minutes.

3. Pour in the Chicken Stock or water and stir to mix well. Raise the heat to high and bring to a boil. Add the salt, pepper, and powdered saffron, if using. Reduce the heat to very low, cover and cook, undisturbed, until the liquid is absorbed and the rice is tender, about 20 minutes.

4. To serve, using a large fork, fluff the rice and gently stir in the parsley. Transfer to a serving bowl.

*Nutritional Analysis
Per Serving:*

CALORIES 173
(KILOJOULES 725)
PROTEIN 3 G
CARBOHYDRATES 28 G
TOTAL FAT 5 G
SATURATED FAT 1 G
CHOLESTEROL 0 MG
SODIUM 292 MG
DIETARY FIBER 1 G

Combined in this satisfying side dish, the lentils and rice together provide a complete source of dietary protein. Basmati rice is a long-grain Indian variety of white rice prized for its distinctive aroma.

LENTIL & RICE PILAF

Serves 4

½ cup (3½ oz/105 g) dried lentils, rinsed
2 tablespoons olive oil
1 small yellow onion, finely chopped
1 garlic clove, peeled and minced
1 cup (7 oz/220 g) basmati rice, rinsed, or long-grain white rice

1¾ cups (14 fl oz/440 ml) Chicken Stock *(recipe on page 127)* or water
½ teaspoon salt
1 tablespoon finely chopped fresh mint
1 tablespoon finely chopped fresh dill
1 tablespoon fresh lemon juice
zest of ½ lemon, cut into strips

Nutritional Analysis Per Serving:

CALORIES 336
(KILOJOULES 1,413)
PROTEIN 13 G
CARBOHYDRATES 57 G
TOTAL FAT 8 G
SATURATED FAT 1 G
CHOLESTEROL 0 MG
SODIUM 440 MG
DIETARY FIBER 4 G

1. Fill a saucepan three-fourths full of water and bring to a boil. Stir in the lentils and boil, uncovered, until almost tender, about 10 minutes. Drain well.

2. In a sauté or large, deep frying pan over medium heat, warm the olive oil. Add the onion and sauté, stirring, until softened, 5–6 minutes. Add the garlic and cook, stirring, for 1 minute longer.

3. Add the rice and the lentils and stir to coat well. Add the Chicken Stock or water and salt and bring to a boil. Reduce the heat to medium-low, cover and cook until the liquid is absorbed, about 15 minutes. Remove from the heat and let stand, covered, for 5 minutes.

4. To serve, add the mint, dill and lemon juice and stir to mix well. Transfer to a serving dish and garnish with the lemon zest.

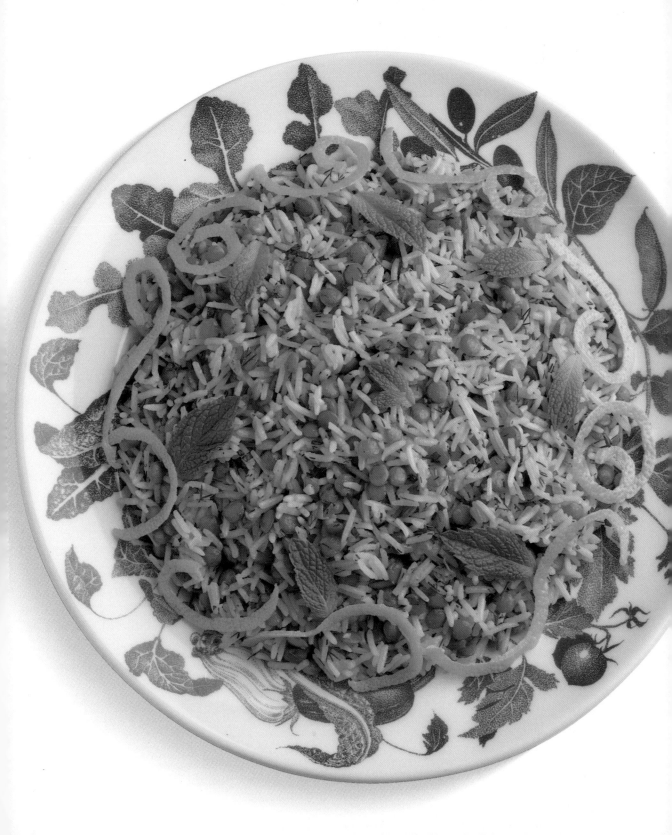

High-fiber brown rice can be a little bit dry and chewy; however, this method turns it into a moist and tender side dish, with vegetables and herbs for flavor. Try it as an accompaniment to grilled turkey burgers or steamed fish.

Mediterranean Brown Rice

Serves 6

4 tablespoons (2 fl oz/60 ml) olive oil
1 leek, green and white parts, finely chopped
2 garlic cloves, peeled and minced
1 teaspoon ground cumin
1 cup (7 oz/220 g) long-grain brown rice
2 cups (16 fl oz/500 ml) water
½ teaspoon salt
¼ teaspoon freshly ground pepper
1 eggplant (aubergine), peeled and cut into cubes
2 ripe tomatoes, peeled, seeded and diced

⅓ cup (2 oz/60 g) crumbled feta cheese
1 tablespoon minced fresh parsley
1 tablespoon finely chopped fresh basil

1. In a sauté or deep frying pan over medium-low heat, warm half the olive oil. Add the leek and cook, stirring occasionally, until softened but not browned, 4–5 minutes. Stir in the garlic and cumin and cook for 30 seconds longer. Add the rice and stir to coat well with the oil. Continue cooking over medium-low heat until the rice begins to color lightly, 3–4 minutes.

2. Pour in the water and stir to mix well. Raise the heat to high and bring to a boil. Add the salt and pepper, reduce the heat to very low, cover and cook, undisturbed, until the rice is tender and the liquid is absorbed, about 40 minutes.

3. Meanwhile, in another sauté or frying pan over medium heat, warm the remaining olive oil. Add the eggplant and sauté, stirring constantly, until just tender, about 10 minutes. Add the tomatoes and continue to sauté, stirring, until all the excess liquid has evaporated, 3–4 minutes.

4. Using a large fork, gently stir the eggplant mixture into the rice mixture. Cover and let stand off the heat for 10 minutes.

5. To serve, transfer to a serving bowl. Using a large fork and being careful not to crush the grains, stir in the feta cheese, parsley and basil.

Nutritional Analysis Per Serving:

Calories 273
(Kilojoules 1,146)
Protein 6 g
Carbohydrates 37 g
Total Fat 12 g
Saturated Fat 3 g
Cholesterol 8 mg
Sodium 302 mg
Dietary Fiber 3 g

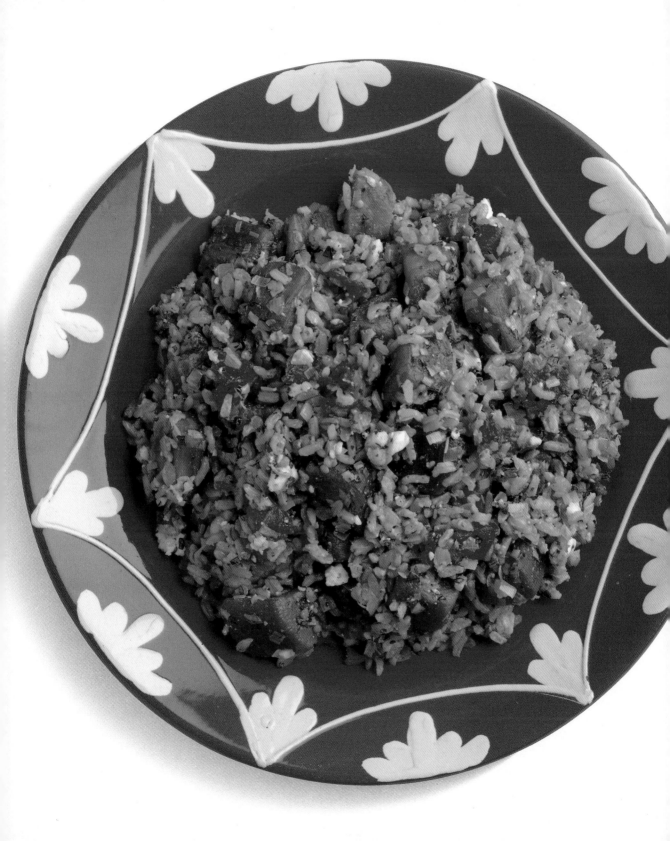

With its rich, nutty flavor and chewy texture, wild rice—not, in fact, a true rice, but the seed of an aquatic grass—goes especially well with poultry or game. Toasting accentuates the flavor of almonds and other nuts (method on page 124).

LONG-GRAIN & WILD RICE PILAF

Serves 4

2 tablespoons olive oil

3 green (spring) onions, green and white parts, finely chopped

6 cups (48 fl oz/1.5 l) water

½ cup (3 oz/90 g) wild rice

½ cup (3½ oz/105 g) long-grain white rice

2 tablespoons slivered almonds, toasted

2 tablespoons golden raisins (sultanas)

½ teaspoon salt

¼ teaspoon freshly ground pepper

1 tablespoon finely chopped fresh parsley

1. In a small frying pan over medium-low heat, warm the olive oil. Add the green onions and sauté, stirring occasionally, until softened, 1–2 minutes.

2. In a saucepan over high heat, bring the water to a boil. Add the wild rice, reduce the heat slightly and simmer, uncovered, for 10 minutes to cook partially.

3. Add the white rice and return to a boil. Cover, reduce the heat to medium-low and cook, undisturbed, until the rices are tender but not mushy and the water is absorbed, about 20 minutes longer.

4. To serve, transfer to a serving bowl, add the sautéed green onions, almonds, raisins, salt, pepper and parsley and stir to mix well.

Nutritional Analysis
Per Serving:

CALORIES 269
(KILOJOULES 1,129)
PROTEIN 6 G
CARBOHYDRATES 41 G
TOTAL FAT 9 G
SATURATED FAT 1 G
CHOLESTEROL 0 MG
SODIUM 279 MG
DIETARY FIBER 2 G

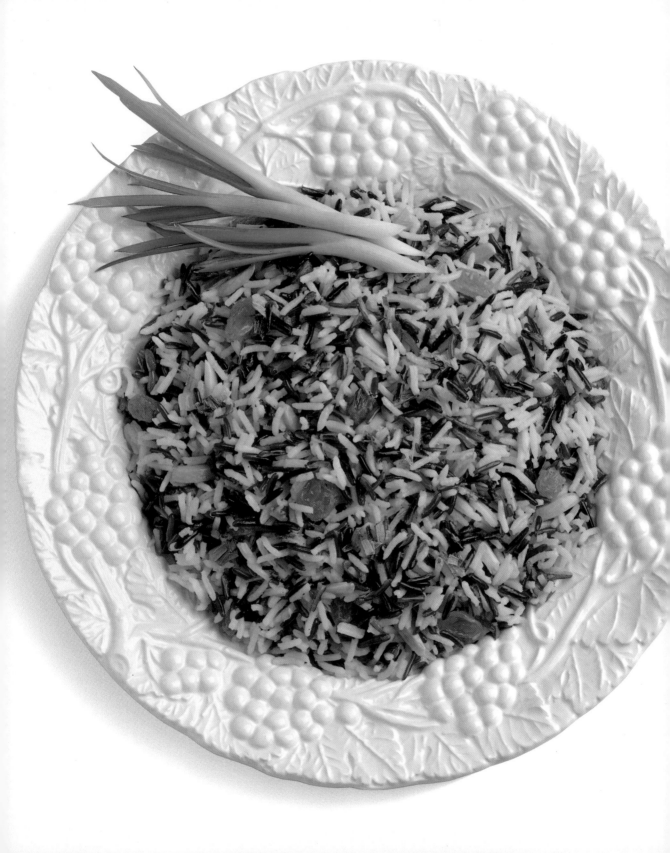

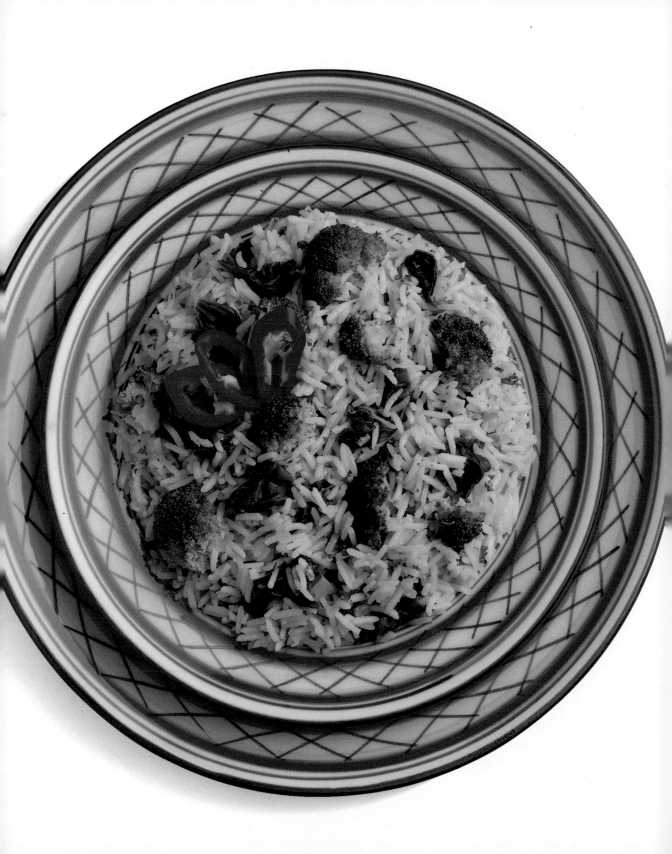

Make this substantial Southwestern-style side dish as mild or spicy as you like simply by adjusting the amount of jalapeño to taste. Serve it with barbecued chicken. Take care to wash your hands and utensils well after working with chilies.

Green Chili Rice

Serves 6

3 tablespoons olive oil
1 yellow onion, finely chopped
1 cup (7 oz/220 g) long-grain white rice
1 small fresh jalapeño pepper, seeded and minced (about 2 teaspoons)
¾ cup (2 oz/60 g) small broccoli florets (from 1 stalk)
2 garlic cloves, peeled and minced

1¾ cups (14 fl oz/440 ml) Chicken Stock *(recipe on page 127)* or water
½ teaspoon salt
½ cup (½ oz/15 g) spinach leaves, coarsely chopped
2 tablespoons finely chopped fresh parsley
1 tablespoon freshly grated Parmesan cheese

1. In a large sauté or deep frying pan over medium heat, warm 2 tablespoons of the olive oil. Add the onion and sauté, stirring occasionally, until lightly browned, 4–5 minutes.
2. Add the rice and stir to coat well. Continue cooking over medium heat until the rice just begins to brown, 3–4 minutes.
3. Stir in the jalapeño, broccoli, garlic, Chicken Stock or water and salt. Stir to mix well. Raise the heat and bring to a boil. Reduce the heat to very low, cover and cook, undisturbed, for 15 minutes.
4. Using a large fork, stir the spinach into the rice. Cover and cook over very low heat until the rice and spinach are tender and the water is absorbed, about 5 minutes longer. Remove from the heat and let stand, covered, for 10 minutes.
5. To serve, gently stir in the remaining 1 tablespoon olive oil, parsley and Parmesan cheese. Transfer to a serving bowl.

Nutritional Analysis Per Serving:

**CALORIES 210
(KILOJOULES 882)
PROTEIN 4 G
CARBOHYDRATES 31 G
TOTAL FAT 8 G
SATURATED FAT 1 G
CHOLESTEROL 1 MG
SODIUM 302 MG
DIETARY FIBER 1 G**

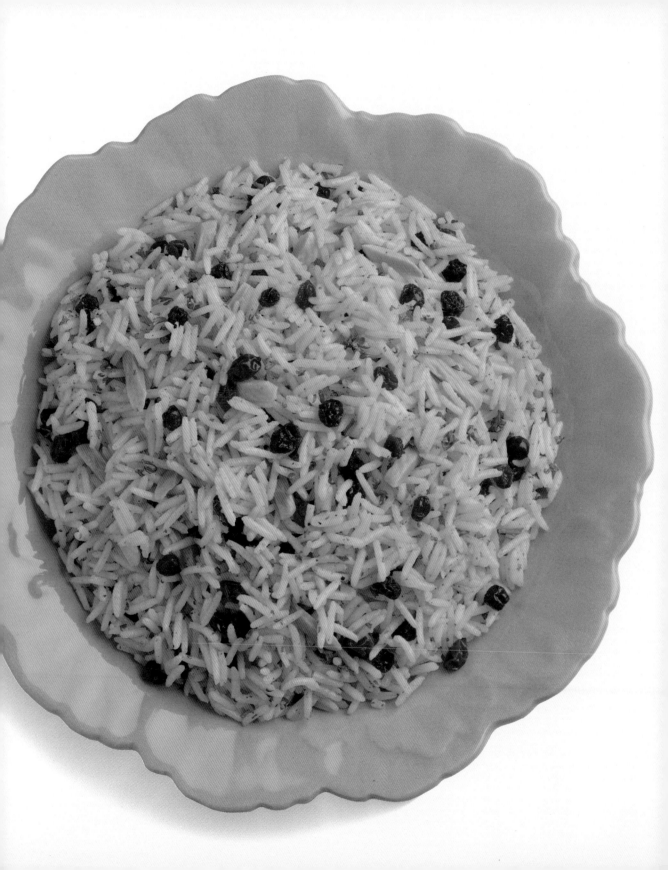

Currants and curry powder impart a Middle Eastern flavor to this side dish, which goes very well with roast chicken, Cornish game hens or braised duck. Find the best curry powder in Indian or Middle Eastern markets.

CURRIED RICE PILAF

Serves 4

1 cup (7 oz/220 g) long-grain
  white rice
2 tablespoons olive oil
1 teaspoon curry powder
½ teaspoon salt
¼ teaspoon freshly ground pepper
1 tablespoon orange juice

2 tablespoons slivered almonds,
  toasted
2 tablespoons dried currants,
  soaked in hot water for 20
  minutes and drained
1 tablespoon finely chopped
  fresh parsley

1. Fill a large saucepan three-fourths full of water, place over medium-high heat and bring to a boil. Add the rice and cook, uncovered, until just tender, about 20 minutes. Drain thoroughly.
2. In a heavy sauté or frying pan over low heat, warm the olive oil. Add the rice, curry powder, salt, pepper, orange juice, almonds and currants. Stir gently until heated through, 1–2 minutes.
3. To serve, gently stir in the parsley. Transfer to a serving bowl.

*Nutritional Analysis
Per Serving:*

**CALORIES 282
(KILOJOULES 1,186)
PROTEIN 5 G
CARBOHYDRATES 45 G
TOTAL FAT 9 G
SATURATED FAT 1 G
CHOLESTEROL 0 MG
SODIUM 277 MG
DIETARY FIBER 1 G**

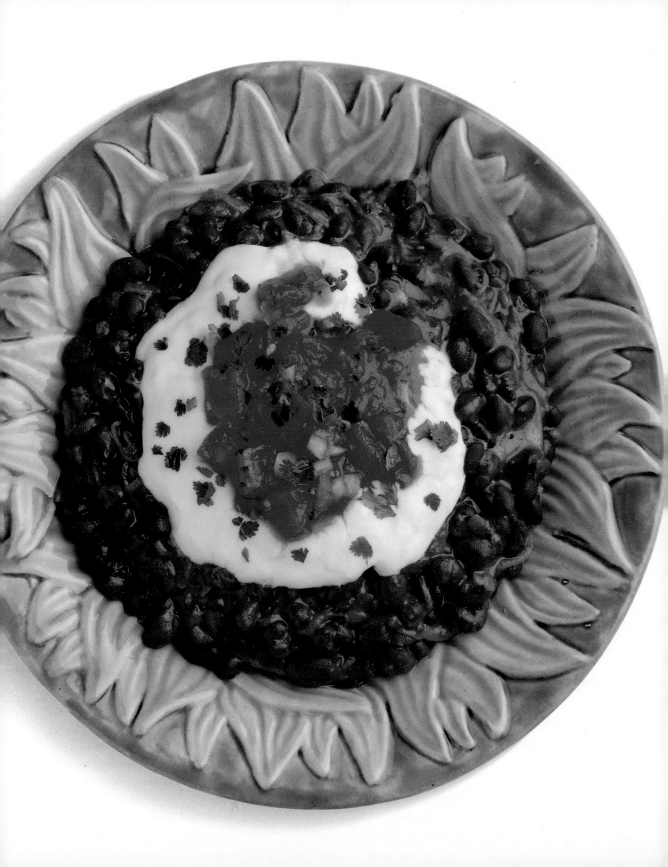

Accompany these slow-cooked beans with warm lowfat corn tortillas, if you like, and serve the combination with grilled poultry, beef or pork for a Mexican-style feast. Or, serve it with chips and cocktails at a party buffet.

Salsa-Topped Spicy Black Beans

Serves 4

1 cup (7 oz/220 g) dried black beans
1 bay leaf
1½ tablespoons olive oil
2 medium or 1 large yellow onion, thinly sliced
2 garlic cloves, peeled and minced
½ small fresh jalapeño pepper, seeded and minced (1 teaspoon)

½ teaspoon ground cumin
2½ tablespoons finely chopped fresh cilantro (fresh coriander)
1 teaspoon salt
⅓ cup (3 fl oz/80 ml) lowfat sour cream
¼ cup (2 fl oz/60 ml) purchased tomato salsa

1. Place the beans in a bowl and add water to cover generously. Soak for at least 3 hours or for as long as overnight. Drain well.
2. In a large saucepan over high heat, place the beans and add cold water to cover generously. Add the bay leaf and bring to a boil. Reduce the heat to low and simmer, uncovered, stirring occasionally, until very tender but not falling apart, 1½–2 hours. The timing will depend upon the age of the beans. Drain the beans, reserving ½ cup (4 fl oz/125 ml) of the liquid.
3. In a sauté or large, deep nonstick frying pan over medium-low heat, warm the olive oil. Add the onions and sauté, stirring, until softened and golden brown, 12–15 minutes. Add the garlic, jalapeño, cumin and 2 tablespoons of the cilantro and cook, stirring, for 1 minute longer.
4. Add the drained beans and reserved cooking liquid and stir to mix thoroughly. Heat until warmed through, 1–2 minutes. Add the salt and stir to mix well.
5. To serve, transfer to a serving bowl. Top with the sour cream, salsa and the remaining ½ tablespoon cilantro.

Nutritional Analysis Per Serving:

CALORIES 278
(KILOJOULES 1,166)
PROTEIN 13 G
CARBOHYDRATES 41 G
TOTAL FAT 7 G
SATURATED FAT 1 G
CHOLESTEROL 5 MG
SODIUM 663 MG
DIETARY FIBER 8 G

Because the cooking time of dried beans varies with their age, there may be excess liquid left when the beans are tender. If so, before you add the Swiss chard, raise the heat and simmer rapidly, uncovered, until the sauce just lightly coats the beans.

Tomatoes, Swiss Chard & White Beans

Serves 6

1½ cups (10½ oz/330 g) dried
  white beans
1½ tablespoons olive oil
3 shallots, finely chopped
1 garlic clove, peeled and minced
2 large plum (Roma) tomatoes,
  ½ lb (250 g) total weight, peeled,
  seeded and finely chopped

3 cups (24 fl oz/750 ml) Chicken
  Stock *(recipe on page 127)* or water
1 small bunch Swiss chard (silverbeet)
½ teaspoon salt
¼ teaspoon freshly ground pepper
1 teaspoon fresh lemon juice
2 tablespoons freshly grated
  Parmesan cheese

*Nutritional Analysis
Per Serving:*

**CALORIES 239
(KILOJOULES 1,004)
PROTEIN 15 G
CARBOHYDRATES 36 G
TOTAL FAT 5 G
SATURATED FAT 1 G
CHOLESTEROL 2 MG
SODIUM 474 MG
DIETARY FIBER 1 G**

1. Place the beans in a bowl and add water to cover generously. Soak for at least 3 hours or as long as overnight. Drain well.
2. In a heavy saucepan over medium-low heat, warm the olive oil. Add the shallots and sauté, stirring, until soft but not brown, about 3 minutes. Add the garlic and sauté for 1 minute longer. Add the tomatoes, Chicken Stock or water and beans. Bring to a boil, reduce heat to low, cover and simmer until the beans are tender but not falling apart, 1–1½ hours.
3. Thinly slice enough of the Swiss chard stems to yield about 1 cup (5 oz/155 g). Tear the leaves into bite-sized pieces. Add the Swiss chard leaves and stems to the beans and stir briefly to mix. Cover and cook over medium-low heat until the chard has wilted slightly, 4–5 minutes. Add the salt, pepper and lemon juice and stir to mix well.
4. To serve, transfer to a serving dish and sprinkle with the Parmesan cheese.

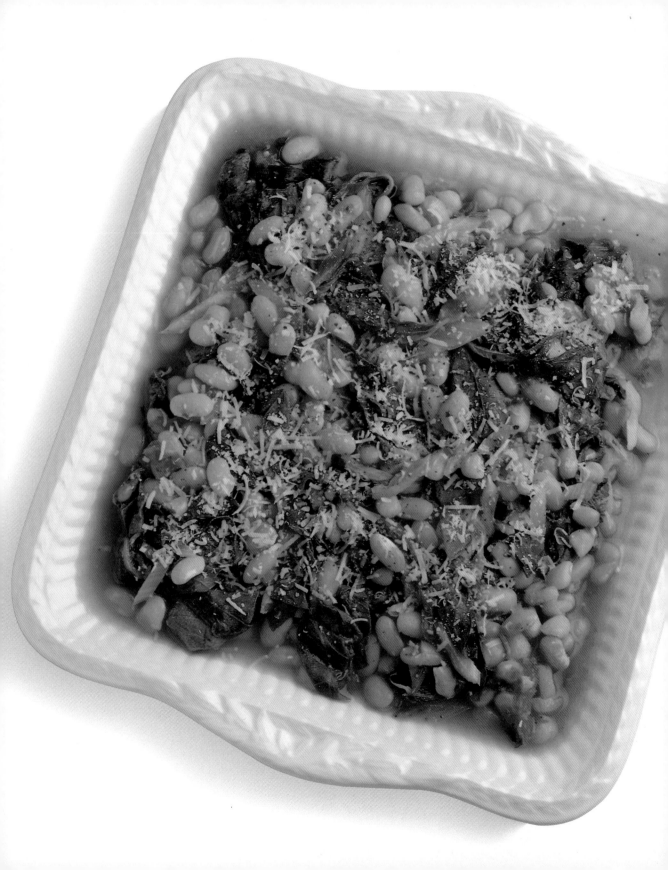

Though it looks like a grain, orzo is in fact a small rice-shaped pasta, available in well-stocked markets and Italian food stores; risi pasta may be substituted. This Mediterranean-style dish goes well with simple grilled veal or chicken.

ORZO & ZUCCHINI

Serves 4

3 zucchini (courgettes), diced
2 tablespoons olive oil
1 large shallot, peeled and finely chopped
½ lb (250 g) fresh white mushrooms, diced
2 garlic cloves, peeled and minced

1 cup (7 oz/220 g) orzo pasta
¼ teaspoon salt
⅛ teaspoon freshly ground pepper
3 tablespoons freshly grated Parmesan cheese
2 tablespoons finely chopped fresh basil

1. Place the zucchini in a clean kitchen towel and wring out all excess moisture.

2. In a sauté or deep frying pan over medium heat, warm the olive oil. Add the shallot and sauté, stirring occasionally, until softened, about 3 minutes. Add the zucchini and continue to sauté until just tender, 3 minutes longer. Add the mushrooms and sauté, stirring, until slightly softened, 2–3 minutes longer. Add the garlic and sauté for 1 minute longer; keep warm.

3. Meanwhile, fill a saucepan three-fourths full of water. Bring to a boil and add the orzo. Cook according to package directions or until al dente, 8–10 minutes. Drain thoroughly.

4. Add the orzo to the vegetable mixture. Cook over medium heat, stirring, until well mixed and heated through, 1–2 minutes. Add the salt and pepper and stir to mix well.

5. To serve, transfer to a serving bowl, add the Parmesan cheese and basil and stir to mix well.

Nutritional Analysis Per Serving:

CALORIES 303
(KILOJOULES 1,271)
PROTEIN 11 G
CARBOHYDRATES 45 G
TOTAL FAT 9 G
SATURATED FAT 2 G
CHOLESTEROL 4 MG
SODIUM 231 MG
DIETARY FIBER 3 G

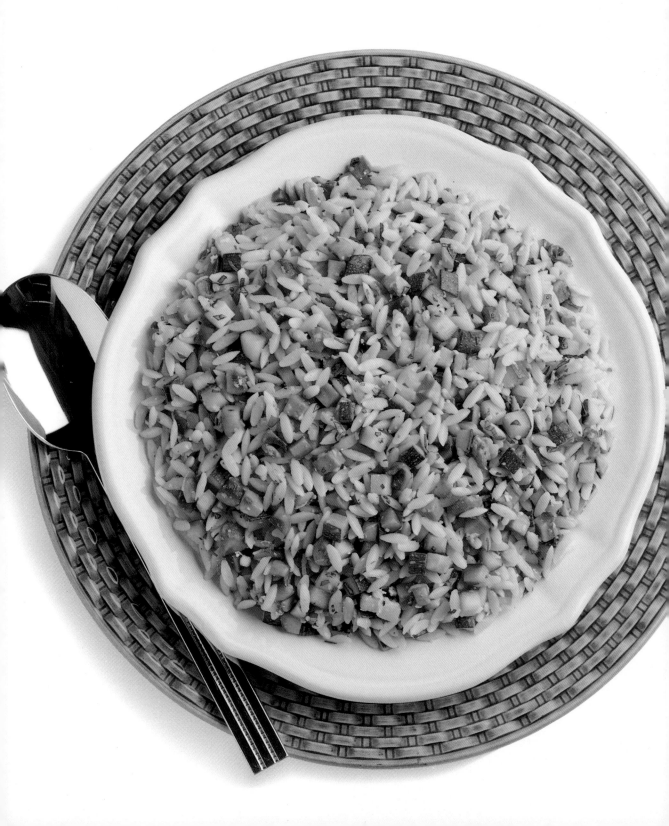

Regular polenta can take up to 45 minutes to cook, but this dish goes together quickly because it uses the widely available instant variety. The fragrant Mixed Herb Pesto makes the cooked Italian-style cornmeal a perfect companion to grilled lamb or veal.

Polenta with Mixed Herb Pesto

Serves 6

2 tablespoons olive oil
2 shallots, peeled and minced
2 green (spring) onions, green and white parts, finely chopped
2 garlic cloves, peeled and minced
7 cups (56 fl oz/1¾ l) Chicken Stock *(recipe on page 127)* or water

2 cups (12 oz/370 g) instant polenta
4 tablespoons (1 oz/30 g) freshly grated Parmesan cheese
½ cup (4 fl oz/125 ml) Mixed Herb Pesto *(recipe on page 127),* at room temperature

1. In a large saucepan over medium heat, warm the olive oil. Add the shallots and sauté, stirring, until softened and just beginning to caramelize, 5–7 minutes. Add the onions and garlic and cook for 1 minute longer, being careful not to brown the garlic.

2. Add the Chicken Stock or water and bring to a boil. Using a measuring cup with a spout, pour in the polenta in a very slow, thin, steady stream, stirring constantly with a wooden spoon. Reduce the heat to medium-low and continue cooking, stirring constantly, until the polenta is very thick, smooth and creamy, about 5 minutes. Add half of the Parmesan cheese and stir it in just until it melts.

3. To serve, spoon the polenta into a serving dish, top with the Mixed Herb Pesto and sprinkle with the remaining Parmesan cheese.

Nutritional Analysis Per Serving:

CALORIES 405
(KILOJOULES 1,699)
PROTEIN 11 G
CARBOHYDRATES 55 G
TOTAL FAT 15 G
SATURATED FAT 3 G
CHOLESTEROL 6 MG
SODIUM 577 MG
DIETARY FIBER 4 G

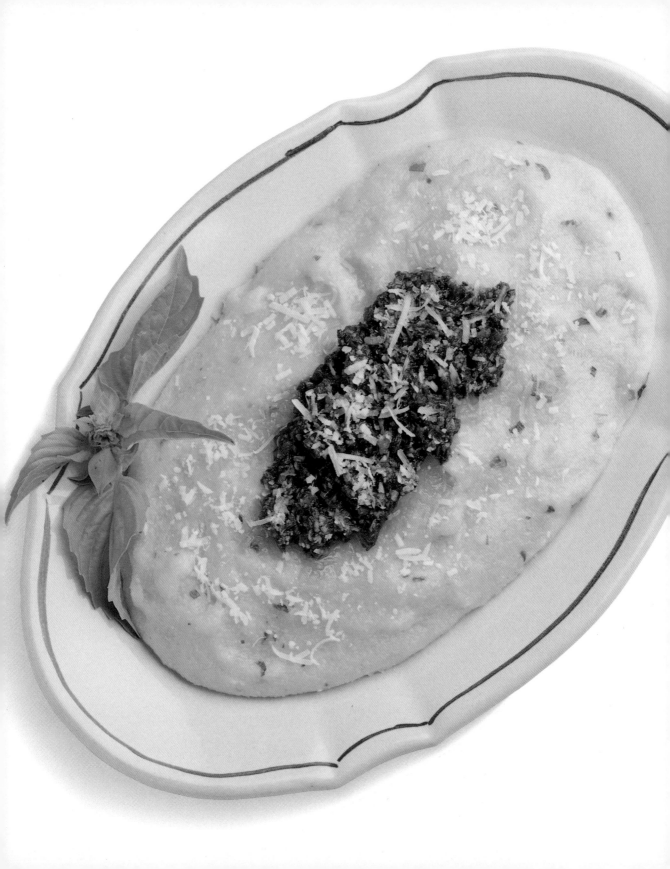

BASIC TERMS & TECHNIQUES

The following entries provide a reference source for this volume, offering definitions of essential or unusual ingredients and providing explanations of fundamental preparation and cooking techniques.

ASPARAGUS

A specialty of springtime, these delicate stalks, whether green or white, slender or plump, sliced or eaten whole, make an excellent side dish.

To Trim Asparagus: Grasp each stalk near its cut end and bend it; the end will snap away at the point where the stalk turns tender. To conserve more of the stalk, however, you can peel away the tough skin near the cut end. Trim the cut end of each stalk; then, using a small, sharp paring knife or vegetable peeler held parallel to the end, thickly cut away the bottom 2 inches (5 cm), gradually cutting more thinly as the skin becomes more tender towards the tip.

BEANS & LENTILS

Beans and lentils provide an important source of protein, fiber and complex carbohydrates; they are also good sources of essential B vitamins and minerals. Before use, dried beans and lentils should be carefully picked over to remove any impurities such as small stones or fibers or any discolored or misshapen beans. Presoak beans in cold water to cover for a few hours to rehydrate them, shorten their cooking time and improve their digestibility; lentils require no presoaking. Rinse canned beans well with cold water to flush out excess sodium.

BEETS

Because the color of these ruby red vegetables bleeds easily into cooking liquids, always cook them before peeling, simmering them completely covered with water until fork-tender, 45–60 minutes for medium-sized beets. Drain and rinse under cold running water until the beets are cool enough to handle; their skins will slip or peel off easily with a small, sharp knife.

BELL PEPPERS

Also known as capsicums, these fresh, sweet-fleshed, bell-shaped members of the pepper family are most common in the unripe green form, although ripened red or yellow varieties are also available. Creamy pale-yellow, orange and purple-black types may also be found.

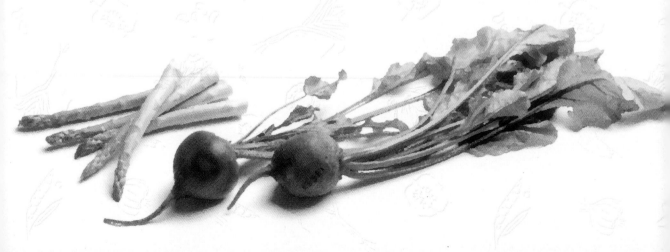

To Prepare a Bell Pepper: Cut the pepper in half lengthwise with a sharp knife. Pull out the stem section from each half, along with the cluster of seeds attached to it. Remove any remaining seeds, along with any thin white membranes, or ribs, to which they are attached. Cut the pepper halves into quarters, strips or thin slices, as called for in the specific recipe.

BREAD CRUMBS

Fresh or dried bread crumbs are sometimes used to contribute body and texture to stuffings or to add a crisp golden topping to baked or broiled side dishes. While bread crumbs may be purchased in food stores, the best-quality and healthiest products will undoubtedly be those you make at home from a good-quality, rustic-style loaf of unbleached wheat bread, with a firm, coarse-textured crumb.

To Make Fresh Crumbs: Cut away the crusts and crumble the bread by hand or in a blender or food processor fitted with the metal blade.

To Make Dried Crumbs: Proceed as for fresh crumbs through crumbling by hand or machine, then spread the crumbs on a baking sheet. Dry slowly, about 1 hour, in an oven set at its lowest temperature. Store in a tightly covered container at room temperature.

BROCCOLI & CAULIFLOWER FLORETS

When a recipe calls for florets of broccoli or cauliflower, simply cut the flowerlike buds or clusters from the ends of the stalks, including about 1 inch (2.5 cm) of stem with each floret. Reserve the stalks for another use.

CABBAGES

The hard, solid cores of green or red cabbages must be cut away before the cabbage can be shredded for cooking.

To Core and Shred Cabbage: Using a knife with a sturdy blade, cut the cabbage in half through its stem end. On each half, cut down at an angle on either side of the core to remove it. (The core may be reserved, to be sliced and boiled, steamed or stir-fried separately.) Turn each half cut side down and, starting at the end opposite the core, cut thin vertical slices to shred.

CHEESES

Although most cheeses are high in fat and therefore largely excluded in large quantities from health-conscious diets, just a little cheese can go a long way to add flavor and richness to healthy side dishes. Cheese is also an excellent source of calcium.

For the best selection and finest quality, buy cheese from a well-stocked food store or delicatessen that offers a wide variety and has a frequent turnover of product. (Also, watch for and sample the reduced-fat cheeses that are now being introduced commercially.) These highly flavored or richly textured cheeses are a good choice when used sparingly in a healthy diet:

CHEDDAR This firm, smooth-textured whole-milk cheese is pale yellow-white to deep yellow-orange. It ranges in taste from mild and sweet when fresh to rich and sharply tangy when aged.

FETA Also called goat cheese, white, salty, sharp-tasting feta cheese is made from sheep's or goat's milk, with a crumbly, creamy-to-dry consistency.

GRUYÈRE A variety of Swiss cheese, gruyère has a firm, smooth texture, small holes and a strong, nutty flavor.

PARMESAN A semi-hard cheese made from half skimmed and half whole cow's milk. Its sharp, salty flavor results from up to two years of aging. In its prime, a good piece of Parmesan cheese is dry but not grainy and flakes easily. For best flavor, purchase versions produced in Italy.

Because of the use of skimmed milk, Parmesan adds significant flavor for its fat content. Buy in block form, to freshly shave or grate as needed, rather than already grated.

RICOTTA A very light, mild Italian cheese made with twice-cooked milk—traditionally sheep's milk, although cow's milk ricotta is far more common. Ricotta is made from the whey left over from making other cheeses, most commonly mozzarella and provolone.

ROMANO Italian variety of cheese traditionally made from sheep's milk, now made from goat's and cow's milk as well. Sold either fresh or, more commonly, aged. The aged form is similar to but notably more tangy than Parmesan. Buy in block form, to freshly shave or grate as needed.

CHILI PEPPERS

The unripened form of any of a wide variety of fresh peppers prized for the mild-to-hot spiciness they impart as a seasoning. They include the mild-to-hot, dark green poblano; the long, mild Anaheim; and the small, fiery jalapeño. When handling any chili, wear kitchen gloves to prevent any cuts or abrasions on your hands from contacting the pepper's volatile oils; wash your hands well with soapy water and take special care not to touch your eyes or any other sensitive areas.

CITRUS ZESTS

The thin outermost layer of a citrus fruit's peel, the zest contains most of its aromatic essential oils, is a lively source of flavor, makes an attractive garnish and contains remarkable amounts of vitamin C.

To Zest Citrus Fruit: Using a zester or hand-held shredder, draw the sharp-edged holes across the fruit's skin to remove the zest in thin strips. Alternatively, using a paring knife or vegetable peeler held almost parallel to the fruit's skin, cut off the zest in thin strips, taking care not to remove any white pith with it, then thinly slice or chop, if desired.

CORN

Before use, fresh sweet corn must be stripped of its green outer husks and the fine inner silky threads must be removed.

To Cut Corn Kernels: If a recipe calls for removing the kernels from an ear of corn, hold the ear by its pointed end, steadying its stalk

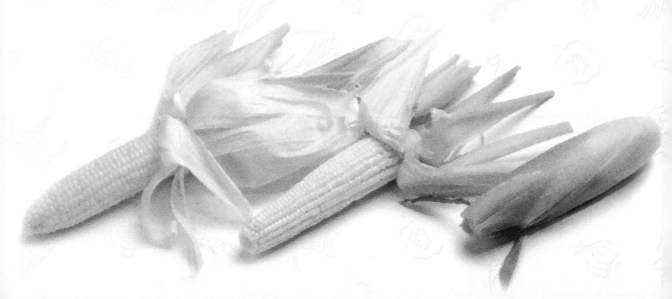

end on a cutting board. Using a sharp, sturdy knife cut down and away from you along the ear, stripping off the kernels. Continue turning the ear with each cut.

CORNSTARCH

This fine, powdery flour ground from the endosperm of corn—the white heart of the kernel—is used as a neutral-flavored thickening agent. Also known as cornflour.

DAIRY PRODUCTS

The rich, mild flavor of milk and milk products can be incorporated into side dishes with little or none of the fat present in whole milk, which contains 3.3 percent fluid fat and thus derives almost half of its calories from fat. Lowfat milk with 2 percent fluid fat, by contrast, gets only 35 percent of its calories from fat; lowfat milk with 1 percent fluid fat has only 23 percent fat calories; and nonfat milk typically derives only 5 percent of calories from fat. Similar percentages also apply to yogurt, which adds tangy enrichment much as sour cream would; seek out, as well, both lowfat and nonfat dairy sour cream, available in well-stocked food stores. Cultured buttermilk, although it has a rich, tangy flavor and thick, creamy texture, is slightly lower in fat than 1 percent lowfat milk, with only 20 percent of calories from fat. Regardless of their fat contents, all dairy products are a primary source of calcium as well as vitamins A and D.

GARLIC

This pungent bulb is popular worldwide as a flavoring ingredient, both raw and cooked. For the best flavor, purchase whole heads of garlic, separating individual cloves from the head as needed. It is best not to purchase more than you will use in 1 to 2 weeks, as garlic can shrivel and lose its flavor with prolonged storage.

To Peel a Garlic Clove: Place on a work surface and cover with the side of a large chef's knife. Press down firmly but carefully on the side of the knife to crush the clove slightly; the dry skin will then slip off easily.

HERBS

Versatile and colorful, culinary herbs add great flavor and visual appeal to side dish recipes and provide an excellent alternative to salt. Keep fresh herbs in water—as you would cut flowers—awaiting use. They will last up to 1 week, if trimmed daily and stored in the refrigerator. Store dried herbs in tightly covered containers in a cool dark place and use within 6 months of purchase.

To Chop Fresh Herbs: Wash the herbs under cold running water and thoroughly shake dry. If the herb has leaves attached along woody stems, pull the leaves from the stems; otherwise, hold the stems together, gather up the leaves into a tight, compact bunch, and use a chef's knife to carefully cut across the bunch to chop the leaves coarsely. Discard the stems.

To Crush Dried Herbs: If using dried herbs, it is best to crush them first in the palm of your hand to release their flavor. Or warm them in a frying pan and crush using a mortar and pestle.

LEEKS

Grown in sandy soil, these leafy-topped, multi-layered vegetables require thorough cleaning.

To Clean a Leek: Trim off the tough ends of the dark green leaves. Trim off the roots. If a recipe calls for leek whites only, trim off the dark-green leaves where they meet the slender pale-green part of the stem. Starting about 1 inch (2.5 cm) from the root end, slit the leek lengthwise. Vigorously swish the leek in a basin or sink filled with cold water. Drain and rinse again; check to make sure that no dirt remains between the tightly packed pale portion of the leaves.

To Slice a Leek: Hold the cleaned leek steadily on a cutting surface and, using a sharp knife, cut crosswise starting at the root end. If a recipe calls for chopped leek, simply chop the slices.

NONSTICK COOKING SPRAY

An aerosol mixture of oil, lecithin (a soybean extract used as an emulsifier), sometimes grain alcohol and a harmless propellant, nonstick cooking sprays coat cooking surfaces, preventing food from sticking and enabling baking or sautéing with little added fat.

NUTS

Because nuts are high in fat they should be avoided in large quantities in a healthy diet, but can be added to recipes in small quantities to contribute their characteristic flavor and texture—as well as vitamins and minerals—with little added fat. Finely ground particles of nuts prepared at home from unsalted shelled nuts allow this to be accomplished easily.

To Toast Nuts: Toasting brings out the full flavor and aroma of nuts. To toast any kind of nut, preheat an oven to 325°F (165°C). Spread the nuts in a single layer on a baking sheet and toast in the oven until they just begin to change color, 5–10 minutes. Remove from the oven and let cool to room temperature. Alternatively, toast nuts in a dry heavy frying pan over low heat, stirring frequently to prevent scorching.

To Chop Nuts: To chop nuts, spread them in a single layer on a nonslip cutting surface. Using a chef's knife, carefully chop the nuts with a gentle rocking motion. Alternatively, put a handful or two of nuts in a food processor fitted with the metal blade and use a few rapid on-off pulses to chop the nuts to desired consistency; repeat with the remaining nuts in batches. Be careful not to process the nuts too long or their oils will be released and the nuts will turn into a paste.

OILS

Although oil is nothing more than a vegetable fat that is liquid at room temperature, and therefore derives 100 percent of its calories from fat, a relatively small amount of oil aids cooking and can add distinctive flavor. Oils are also an excellent source of vitamin E and play an essential role in transporting the fat-soluble vitamins in our diet. Vegetable oils contain no cholesterol.

Store all oils in tightly covered containers in a cool, dark place.

OLIVE OIL With its rich flavor and range of culinary uses, olive oil deserves its reputation as the queen of edible oils. Medical studies show that monounsaturated fat, which is found in olive oil, may reduce the risk of heart disease, cancer and diabetes when used in a lowfat diet. Olive oils are identified by their acidity. Extra-virgin olive oil is the finest. Its low acidity makes it smooth on the palate when used in uncooked dishes or added to hot dishes at the end of cooking. Both virgin and pure olive oil have slightly higher acidity levels and are fine for cooked dishes.

VEGETABLE & SEED OILS Use flavorless vegetable and seed oils such as safflower, corn and canola (rapeseed) for their high cooking temperatures and bland flavors.

PASTA

The growing popularity of pasta has resulted in an ever wider range of choices. All pasta, whether fresh or dried, can be prepared as carbohydrate-rich side dishes. Cook as directed below, drain and mix with a healthy topping such as chopped fresh herbs and a drizzle of olive oil; sautéed chopped fresh tomatoes and basil; or a few spoonfuls of Mixed Herb Pesto (page 127).

To Cook Pasta: To cook any pasta perfectly al dente—tender but still chewy—use enough boiling water to let the pasta circulate freely;

salting the water is not necessary. Cook 2 to 3 ounces of pasta per person as a side dish. Cooking time depends on the shape, size and dryness, with fresh pasta generally taking 1–3 minutes and dried 3–15 minutes. Check suggested times on packaging and test for doneness by removing a piece, letting it cool briefly and eating it.

POLENTA

Italian term for a cooked mush of coarsely ground cornmeal. In most cases, instant polenta—available in well-stocked food stores and Italian delicatessens—may be used instead of the old-fashioned, long-simmered variety.

POMEGRANATES

Autumn fruit of Persian origin, pomegranates are shaped like a large orange, with leathery red skin concealing hundreds of bright ruby-red seeds about the size and shape of small corn kernels. The seeds are composed largely of a juicy, sweet pulp and can be eaten on their own, used as a colorful garnish, or squeezed to yield a juice that becomes a sweet, aromatic flavoring in its own right.

To Remove Pomegranate Seeds: With a sharp, serrated knife, thinly slice off the stem end of the fruit to expose the seeds. Then, score the fruit's leathery skin top to bottom and peel it off. Use a small spoon or a fork to scrape out the seeds, taking care not to crush them; discard any pieces of the white membrane that separates the sections of seeds.

RICE

Rice purchased in bulk may need to be rinsed prior to cooking to remove added talc. Most packaged rice does not require rinsing.

To Cook Rice: Allow 2 cups of water for every cup of uncooked white rice. Bring the water to a boil and add the rice; when the water returns to a boil, reduce the heat to very low, cover and cook, without uncovering, until all the water has been absorbed and the rice is tender—about 20 minutes for long-grain white rice. Unpolished brown rice retains more fiber and nutrients, including B vitamins, than white rice. Because it still has the bran, brown rice needs to be cooked slightly longer and with more water than white rice.

SHALLOTS

These small members of the onion family have brown skins, white-to-purple flesh and taste like a cross between sweet onion and garlic—making them a versatile seasoning in side dishes.

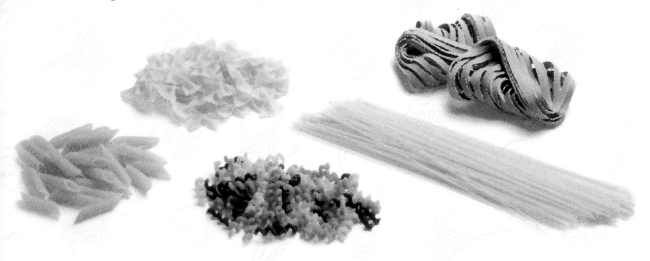

SPINACH

Because this leafy vegetable is grown in sandy soil, it requires careful washing to eliminate all dirt and sand.

To Stem and Wash Spinach: To remove tough stems from mature leaves, fold the leaf in half, glossy side in. Grasp the stem and pull it toward the leaf tip, peeling it off the leaf. In a sink or large basin filled with cold water to cover, agitate the leaves in the water to remove their dirt. Then lift the leaves out of the water and set aside. Drain the sink or basin thoroughly and rinse out all dirt and sand. Repeat the procedure until no grit remains.

TOMATOES

Recipes in which fresh tomatoes are to be cooked sometimes call for removing peels and seeds.

To Peel Tomatoes: Bring a saucepan of water to a boil. Using a small, sharp knife, cut out the core from the stem end of the tomato. Then cut a shallow X in the skin at the tomato's base. Submerge for about 20 seconds in the boiling water, then remove and dip in a bowl of cold water. Starting at the X, peel the skin from the tomato, using your fingertips and, if necessary, the knife blade. Cut the tomatoes in half and turn each half cut-side down. Then cut as directed in the individual recipes.

To Seed a Tomato: Cut the tomato in half crosswise. Squeeze gently to force out the sacs of seeds.

VINEGARS

Literally "sour wine," vinegar results when certain strains of yeast cause wine—or some other alcoholic liquid such as sherry, apple cider or Japanese rice wine—to ferment for a second time, turning it acidic.

The best-quality wine vinegars begin with good-quality wine. Red wine vinegar, like the wine from which it is made, has a more robust flavor than vinegar produced from white wine. Balsamic vinegar, a specialty of Modena, Italy, is a vinegar made from reduced grape juice and aged for many years. Flavored vinegars are made by adding herbs such as tarragon and dill or fruits such as raspberries to wine vinegar.

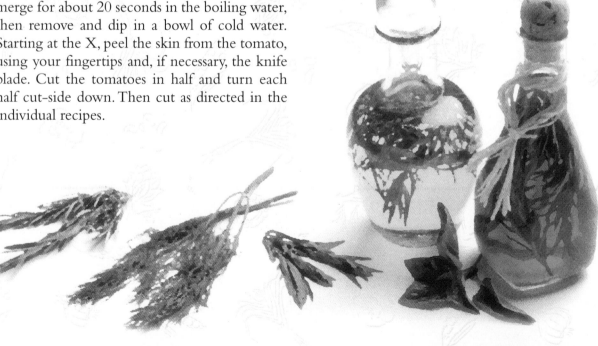

BASIC RECIPES

The following recipes provide a healthy base for many recipes used throughout this volume. Both can be made ahead and stored.

MIXED HERB PESTO

This lively herb paste enhances vegetable, potato and rice dishes as well as traditional pasta. For the finest results, select the freshest herbs available.

Makes 1 cup (8 fl oz/250 ml)

2 garlic cloves, peeled
2 cups (2 oz/60 g) fresh basil leaves (about 1 bunch)
¼ cup (⅓ oz/10 g) fresh parsley leaves
⅓ cup (1 oz/30 g) sliced green (spring) onions
1 tablespoon minced fresh rosemary or
  2 teaspoons dried rosemary
1 tablespoon fresh thyme leaves or 2 teaspoons
  dried thyme
⅓ cup (3 fl oz/80 ml) olive oil
¼ teaspoon salt
¼ teaspoon freshly ground pepper
½ cup (2 oz/60 g) freshly grated Parmesan
  cheese

1. In a food processor fitted with the metal blade, process the garlic cloves until finely chopped.
2. Add the basil, parsley, green onions, rosemary and thyme and process until puréed.
3. With the blades turning, slowly pour the olive oil in a thin, steady stream. Add the salt, pepper and Parmesan cheese and process until well blended.
4. If not using immediately, store in a tightly covered container in the refrigerator for up to 1 week or freezer for several months.

Per 1 Tablespoon Serving: Calories 61 (Kilojoules 255), Protein 2 g, Carbohydrates 2 g, Total Fat 5 g, Saturated Fat 1 g, Cholesterol 2 mg, Sodium 92 mg, Dietary Fiber 0 g

CHICKEN STOCK

Using a good-quality chicken stock when cooking adds a dimension of flavor not found in water alone.

Makes about 8 cups (64 fl oz/2 l)

3 lb (1.5 kg) chicken necks and backs
2 celery stalks
2 carrots, peeled
1 yellow onion, halved
1 leek, green and white parts, sliced
1 fresh parsley stem
1 bay leaf
1 fresh thyme sprig
1 teaspoon salt

1. In a 3-qt (3-l) saucepan, combine the chicken pieces, celery, carrots, onion and leek. Place the parsley stem, bay leaf and thyme sprig on a small square of cheesecloth (muslin). Bring the corners together, tie securely with kitchen string and add to the pan. Add water to cover generously. Place, uncovered, over medium heat and slowly bring to a boil.
2. Reduce the heat to low and simmer, uncovered, for 3 hours, occasionally skimming off any scum that forms on the surface. Add water, as needed.
3. Add the salt and stir to mix well. Line a colander with cheesecloth (muslin) and place over a large bowl. Strain the stock through the lined colander. Remove and discard the contents of the colander. Let the stock cool, cover and refrigerate until the fat solidifies on top. Using a large spoon, remove and discard the fat from the surface.
4. If not using the stock immediately, store in tightly covered containers in the refrigerator for up to 3 days or freezer for up to 4 months.

Per 1 Cup Serving: Calories 30 (Kilojoules 127), Protein 2 g, Carbohydrates 3 g, Total Fat 1 g, Saturated Fat 0g, Cholesterol 0mg, Sodium 322 mg, Dietary Fiber 0g

INDEX